W9-AIP-964

The Complete Herbal Handbook
for the Dog and Cat

by the same author

THE ILLUSTRATED HERBAL HANDBOOK
FOR EVERYONE

THE COMPLETE HERBAL HANDBOOK
FOR FARM AND STABLE

CATS NATURALLY

The Complete Herbal Handbook for the Dog and Cat

Juliette de Baïracli Levy

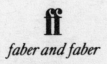

faber and faber

First published in 1955
under the title *The Complete Herbal Book for the Dog*
by Faber and Faber Limited
3 Queen Square London WC1N 3AU
Second edition, 1963
Third edition, 1971
Fourth edition, 1975
Fifth edition, under new title, 1985
Sixth edition, 1991
Reprinted with corrections 1992

Photoset by Parker Typesetting Service Leicester
Printed and bound in Great Britain by Mackays of Chatham PLC

All rights reserved

© Juliette de Baïracli Levy, 1955, 1963, 1971, 1975, 1985, 1991, 1992

Juliette de Baïracli Levy is hereby identified as author of this work
in accordance with Section 77 of the Copyright, Designs and Patents Act
1988.

*This book is sold subject to the condition that it shall not, by way of trade
or otherwise, be lent, resold, hired out or otherwise circulated without the
publisher's prior consent in any form of binding or cover other than that
in which it is published and without a similar condition including this
condition being imposed on the subsequent purchaser*

A CIP record for this book is available from the British Library
ISBN 0–571–16115–4

10

TO

MY TURKUMAN AFGHAN HOUNDS

who have wonderfully justified my belief in herbal medicine
and Nature method of canine rearing. Who have never
known disease and whose names, such as Turkuman Bam-
boo, Turkuman Pomegranate, Turkuman Dammar Pine-tree,
Turkuman Wild Kashmiri Iris, Champion Turkuman Camel-
thorn, and that of her son, American Champion Turkuman
Nissim's Laurel, in the opinion of fellow Afghan breeders will
live on in Afghan pedigrees for ever.

My special thanks, in this new sixth edition, to those Afghans
who travelled the world with me, guarding me valiantly in
lonely places during my endless search for herbal lore: Fuego
(The Great), Saraband, Tullipan, Cingane, Esparto-grass,
Donna, Cinderella (skilled killer of rats!) and her son Kaftan
(The Wise), and Kaftan's son Lad-lad (extraordinary catcher
of rabbits), all of Turkuman.

And now for the sixth edition of this book, updating the
Turkumans:

Tyeish (The Wizard), judged greatest male Afghan of all
Greece, son of Lad-lad.

And from Tyeish's mate, Yanshoof (the Very Beloved), Owli
(The Winged-footed) and her daughter Cuckoo Viyah (The
Huntress) whose kill of rats has equalled that of her ancestor
Cinderella, and also from Owli, two special sons, Kabul (King
Kabul) beauty and racing champion, and Dolphin (The
Mighty). Dolphin's mate Flute (The Loving-one) direct
descendant, third generation, from The Royal Kennel of
Afghanistan, has given me Clair-de-Lune (The Queen) silver-
white, my most beautiful Afghan hound ever.

IMPORTANT NOTE FOR READERS IN GREAT BRITAIN

Since this book was written, the natural habitat of many wild plants has disappeared and some herbs have become rare in the wild because of building developments, intensive farming, and other pressures on land use.

In an effort to prevent these rare plants from extinction, the Wildlife and Countryside Act 1981 and its Variation of Schedule Order 1988 make it an offence for any unauthorized person to pick, uproot, destroy or offer for sale almost a hundred wild plants in Great Britain.

It is also an offence for an unauthorized person to *uproot any wild plant*, whether or not it is on the protected list.

The author strongly advises readers to grow their own herbs or obtain dried herbs from health food shops.

The Wildlife and Countryside Act 1981 and the Wildlife and Countryside Act (Variation of Schedule) Order 1988 can be obtained through HMSO bookshops. Alternatively, a list of the fully protected plant species can be obtained from the Department of the Environment, Tollgate House, Houlton Street, Bristol, BS2 9DJ.

Readers in countries other than Great Britain should check local regulations before gathering flowers in the wild.

Contents

CONTENTS

Foreword

THE DOG AND CAT, AMAZING SELF-TAUGHT HERBALISTS

As a beginning I shall tell that the Greek god of medicine, Asclepius, declared that of all the creatures it was the dog which he admired most, because the dog knew and used herbs to prevent and cure all the ailments of the canine race. The cat, to a lesser degree, shares this knowledge. (The god Asclepius is always shown with a walking staff around which is twined his constant companion, a snake.) The snake I have well observed is also a useful herbalist, eating many leafy things which have beneficial medicinal properties. I have had pet snakes in my gardens and I share Asclepius's love for them.

When I see my Afghan hounds in my gardens, or in the fields, or along the river-sides or sea-shores of the many lands where we have been together, I am always amazed at the way they have their selected medicinal plants, shrubs and trees, and know where to find them and how to use them. By use, I mean the amount to be eaten to serve its purpose. Mostly their use is as a laxative or to promote vomiting, and they know exactly how much to achieve one or the other effect.

My Afghan hounds' list of herbs is as follows (many of these herbs are also used by foxes and cats).

The favourite dog medicine, also much eaten by cats, is *couch grass*. This grass is so much a first choice of dogs that its botanical name is *Agrospyron canina* (*canis* is dog). Of this herb they eat the leaves *and* the root, which they either vomit up, with much yellow bile fluid, or excrete. It is a cleanser of the bowels and for removal of worms. When my dogs cannot get couch grass they will utilize other grasses, but do so with reluctance. Their next choice after couch grass seems to be wild oats.

Of the non-grassy plants, a favourite is cleavers (goose-grass); they eat this as a food as well as a medicine. Cleavers is the herb richest in copper which is probably why they choose it. They also utilize dandelion, lemon-grass, fumitory, wood-sage, fennel, mustard (leaves and flowers), strawberry and borage. Their eating of the last-named herb is so persistent that I have to keep many of my borage plants safely out of reach of my hounds or they would eat the lot! Also chosen are garlic (the leaves, especially the thin-leaved type), bramble leaves (despite their prickly nature), mulberry leaves (in quantity), fig leaves (in small amounts). The choice of fig leaves is really remarkable as they contain a white, caustic juice which is very burning. Yet I expect this caustic juice is what the hounds seek, as they very soon either vomit up the leaves or, later, excrete them.

With all this herbal knowledge instinctive to the dog and, to a lesser degree, to the cat, it is indeed sad that dogs and cats today, often kept in enclosures in which all vegetation is soon spoilt by trampling or by soiling with urine and faeces, cannot get their vital herbs fresh from the earth and have to rely on dried prepared herbs from the pharmacist. Herbs can, however, be planted in pots and do well grown in that way. The pots must be placed high enough so that the dogs cannot urinate on them and thus kill them.

Our dogs should be taught to eat the highly beneficial figs;

in dried form they are most enjoyed, but remove the hard stem stumps. Figs are rich in vitamins and minerals as well as being internally cleansing. I feed dried figs to my Afghans usually five days in the week – three or four figs is the usual amount per day.

Cats have a special choice in a variety of *mint* known as catnip or cat-mint. They eat it and also roll in it (with joy!). The rolling might be a skin and hair tonic, but it is also a possible disguise of cat scent when they are hunting prey, catnip being a very pungent herb.

Finally, it is interesting to relate that, having bred my Turkuman Afghans over fifty years, it is my present-day Afghans which are by far my cleverest and most ardent herbalists. I attribute this to the Bell-Murray type, which is now strong in my Turkuman ancestry through a hound (beautiful, almost coatless), Lazar de Champnol (from Branwen). The Bell-Murrays were direct out of Afghanistan, not inbred with other hounds from other lands, and Afghanistan is a great herbal land. Lazar's daughter, Turkuman Branwen Fleur d'Afghan, was the first of my Afghans to eat fig leaves. Her daughter, Turkuman Flame Azalea d'Afghan (coatless) exquisite and true Bell-Murray, ate fig leaves and taught us newly the eating of the important herb, cleavers, fresh from the hedgerow. And her daughter (coated, not Bell-Murray type, but of Bell-Murray breeding) is with me now and my best herbalist ever, using all the herbs I have listed and teaching me newly: strawberry leaves as an emetic and the tubers of Jerusalem artichokes for prevention of stones in kidneys. I managed (difficult) to race indoors and get my camera in time to catch her eating fig leaves from the tree.

Margaret Niblock, England's leading breeder of Afghan hounds and author (see Recommended Books list), gives me the following information of Afghans as herbalists, and this of course applies to all other breeds of dog, as verified by Asclepius.

My Khanabad Afghans also eat goosegrass, but most interesting of all they are crazy about silage! I *must* try and get a photo, like you have done with your 'fig leaves eater' as positive proof. It is hilarious, but as soon as a bag of silage is opened to give to our cattle, horse and donkey, the dogs hasten to grab mouthfuls of the stuff and gobble it up. It is made from cuttings of the orchard grass, mixed herbage (NO fertilizers or additives used, of course). This makes wonderful silage which we put into strong plastic bags (of dust-bin type) and compress as hard as possible to get out all the air, and then leave it for at least eight weeks to seep and settle.

I consider that this from Margaret Niblock is a good tip for others with orchards and a number of dogs, to make silage as a health food supplement.

Back to cats: Sarah Gleadell, of Faber and Faber (publishers of my herbal books) writes me, aptly.

As you know I have three, half-Abyssinian cats. Our lawn patch consists almost entirely of couch-grass, you will be glad to hear. Maybe that is why our cats are so healthy. They come and go entirely as they please and if they are poorly they just rest up for a couple of days and then get going again. But they are hardly ever ill.

That is that. Bravo!

Introduction

The Complete Herbal Handbook for the Dog and Cat combines all my previous canine herbal works, together with much new material which I have been collecting on my world travels since 1947. I first had published three paperback canine herbals in the mid 1930s; and it was the first of these books, *The Cure of Canine Distemper*, which established the then absolutely unknown herbal work in the canine world and attracted to herbal medicine many of England's greatest breeders who, to this day over fifty years later, are following and advocating herbal treatments as keenly as ever.

My puppy-rearing book, *Puppy Rearing by Natural Methods*, was published in England in 1947 and proved so popular that it went into three editions within the year. It was the first of my canine books to achieve foreign translation, being published by Albert Müller, of Zurich, and my other paperbacks followed there later, in beautifully bound editions. All three books were considered worthy of translation by veterinary professors: *Puppy Rearing*, translated by Dr Eugene Sieferle, Zurich; *Medicinal Herbs: Their Use in Canine Ailments*, translated by Dr H. Graf, Veterinary Pharmacology Institute of Zurich University; *Canine Distemper*, translated by F. Granderath, Doctor of Medicine and Veterinary Surgery, Berlin. The puppy-rearing book has achieved eight editions.

My travels in search of authentic and original herbal treatments have been the basis of all my herbal work, and the travels continue. I have covered much of North America and Mexico and, more recently, Turkey, Austria and Israel; also Greece where I have now lived for some years. I agree very much with the opinion of the great herbalist and doctor of medicine of the Middle Ages, Theophrastus Paracelsus von Hohenheim, usually known as Paracelsus. He urges his students to travel in search of medical knowledge and experience, and he himself travelled in many lands, learning mostly from peasants and wandering gypsies. He, in time, became healer to kings and princes, for with the knowledge that he had acquired he cured diseases no other doctor was able to cure. Paracelsus taught: 'The knowledge to which we are entitled is not confined within the limits of our own country, and does not run after us, but waits until we go in search of it. No one becomes master of practical experience in his own house, neither will he find a teacher of the secrets of Nature in the corners of his own room.'

The 'secrets of Nature' are known to all wild creatures and on these they thrive. I have a beloved tame hawk which responds equally well to Natural Rearing and herbal treatments as do bees! I raise bees which are prized for their good health and resistance to disease, and also for their rich honey.

Herbal medicine has grown as the herbs themselves, which are spread over the face of the earth, healthful and ineradicable. For this medicine has clean roots, free of all commercial exploitation of animals and, above all, it is part of Nature's own all-wise teachings.

There are many people to whom the idea of using herbs (which can be bought dried, or otherwise skilfully prepared, by those who cannot gather them wild, as I do) to treat the ailments of their dogs appears nonsensical, or impossible. Yet my previous canine herbals, first published at my own expense because of the prejudices of orthodox veterinary medicine, have sold in their thousands. They have not sold because of any literary merit or appeal to those who buy a herbal book for 'quaint' country lore and 'amusing' extracts from old works; they have sold because every book has meant cures in a widening circle of success, convincing orthodox veterinary surgeons throughout Europe and America.

The few letters from dog owners and breeders which I have found space for in this book, are not included as testimonials for patent medicines; they are the supporting evidence for my unorthodoxy. They mean that these writers, and hundreds more for whom I have no space, who tried my cures with scepticism, have saved their dogs from suffering and death, and have written in gratitude. Spread over a fifty-year period, covering all breeds and representing all classes of dog owner, they are better evidence for the success of my methods than can be shown by many manufacturers of chemicals sold by the shallow magic of advertising.

I would say to all dog owners whose prejudices are aroused by my opinions and my ideas, or even my literary style: please ignore me; it is not what I think that matters – it is your dog. Give him a chance and try my herbal treatments when science fails; if possible, give him a better chance by trying herbs before it may be too late.

Distemper, hard pad, parvovirus, mange, and many other newer diseases, destroy hundreds of pets and show dogs every year, because the vet called in by the trusting owner frequently says that nothing can be done, for he will not try herbal remedies that have stood the test of countless centuries in many countries. I ask you neither to believe me nor to condemn my treatments until you have tried them. My purpose in writing this book is to save your dog, who should not be denied his chance of Nature's remedies by the prejudices of his owners.

It is ironical that when there is a universal revival in herbs, with such big powers as Russia, the People's Republic of

China, and India, by command of their rulers restoring their ancient heritage of herbal remedies, and while furthermore this is THE MEDICINE for MANKIND as ordained in the Bible, the ruling veterinary body of the UK is trying to ban the use of many of the long and well-proved herbs – such great ones as comfrey, sage and poppy. The findings are based on unnatural tests made on laboratory rats, huge amounts of the 'tested' herb being forced upon them through arranged hunger. Herbs will survive this as they have survived other troubles in the past.

I must here register my thanks to the breeders, great and small, who have pioneered my canine herbal treatments throughout the world: to Professor Dr Edmond Bordeaux Szekely and the late Sir Albert Howard, for their interest and encouragement in the early years; to Richard de la Mare, of Faber & Faber, my publishers in England, for his endless personal help and encouragement; to the late Arthur Marples, Editor of *Our Dogs* journal, England, who described my herbal work as 'important' as long ago as 1935, when it was a tiny and weak seed, and gave me so much space to speak freely for herbs in his important journal. Also my thanks go to the late Leo C. Wilson, FZS, international judge, journalist, and editor of *Dog World*, England, who constantly supported my work despite the attacks he had to face thereby; to P.R. Moxon of *The Shooting Times*, the great gun-dogs expert and author who, calling my herbal book his 'canine Bible', has spread far its teachings; and to P.M.C. Toepel, international judge, of Holland, for his kind foreword to the Dutch edition of my canine herbal.

I want also to declare my thanks to people (whose names come immediately to mind) among the many great dog breeders and judges who supported my work and therefore made it possible for me to withstand orthodox veterinary opposition: Kathleen Barker, author and canine artist; Betty

Butterworth, USA; Dora Clarke; Viscountess Chelmsford; Catherine Drinkwater, journalist; Thelma Gray; the Duchess of Hamilton; Ethelwyn Harrison, USA; the Hutchinsons of Helaugh; Sol Malkin, editor and publisher, USA; the Duchess of Montrose; Douglas Oliff; Ann and Bill Petty, Canada; Lady Marjorie Pryse; Lady Kitty Ritson, Lady Rose; Edith Schniewind, Germany; Sunny Shay, USA; the Walker sisters, USA; Mrs M.K. Wentworth-Smith and Mrs Wingfield Digby.

PART ONE

Natural Rearing
of Dogs and Cats

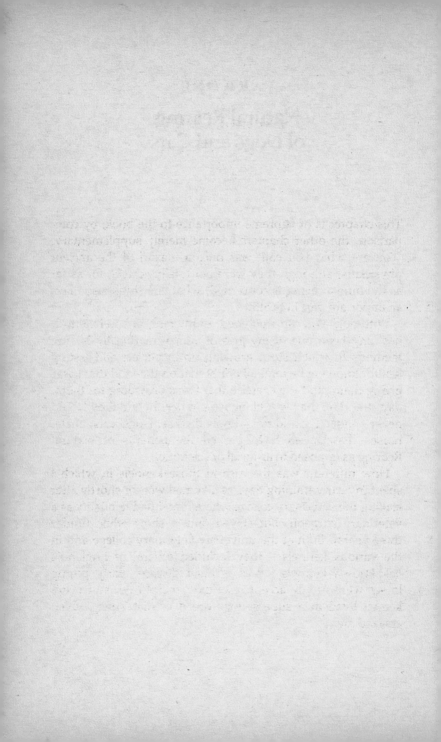

1

Diet for Dogs

This chapter is of supreme importance to the book; by comparison, the other chapters become merely supplementary. 'You are what you eat!' was once a maxim of the ancient physicians, although they were not totally correct; for as far as the human being is concerned, what you think also plays an important part in health.

With dogs you can feed good, indifferent, or bad health. It has long been one of my joys of animal rearing by Nature methods to watch stock growing up in perfect and lasting health, knowing beyond all doubt that on the food that I was giving them, and the exercise that I was providing for them, day after day, they would increase in health, and they would never – indeed, could not – know disease. Dogs, cats, goats, horses, hawks, all have proved the benefits of Natural Rearing as opposed to artificial or scientific.

How different was the case in those kennels in which I spent my early training days as a kennel worker shortly after leaving the veterinary college where I intended to qualify as a veterinary surgeon, but stayed only a short while (under three years). Both at the university veterinary college and in the various kennels – they included several of England's best-known kennels – I saw much disease. Early puppy losses were calmly accepted as the general rule, and every kennel lived in a superstitious dread of distemper, which amazed me.

It seemed to me so completely wrong, this acceptance of inevitable disease: why should all domestic animals, as well as human children, be so afflicted with disease, while other creatures – for example, wild birds – remain almost totally immune? Surely the root cause lay in the hands of man? Man caused disease, inflicted this unnatural state upon everything which came under his unhappy domination, from animal to plant. I soon began to admire everything that was wild: the shining health of wild ponies and wild deer which I met with in the uninhabited parts of Europe, where I used to stay whenever possible, always inspired me, as did the health of the wild plants in contrast to the cultivated ones. I have never found blight on a wild rose: but just think of, and contrast them with, cultivated roses, which frequently suffer a multitude of diseases. To keep my own life and the life of all animals in my care – dogs, cats, goats, horses – as close as possible to Nature then became a campaign of paramount importance to me; and the resultant good health of my animals, my children and myself has been sufficient reward for any trouble involved.

That is the first and supreme law of healthful puppy and kitten rearing, a natural life and a diet of natural foods. The natural life will be fully dealt with in the chapter on general care of puppies; this chapter is primarily concerned with diet.

Although diet is referred to in other chapters of this book, I should like to deal with it fully now, keeping in mind always that it rests in the hands of the human owners as to whether an animal is to live its full life span in true and total health, or to be cut off by disease in early infanthood, or to live a miserable life of subhealth. Food has a threefold purpose for the consumer: to nourish, to induce growth and to give health protection. Dr Howard Schneider, PhD, asks: 'Can we promote resistance to infectious disease by diet? Here is a subject which never languishes for discussion.' This herbal

4

book will help to prove that natural diet has a very large and effective influence on disease prevention.

MEAT FEEDING

The dog is of the Carnivora order and he was a flesh-eating beast in his wild state. Well-preserved skeletons of wild or semi-wild dogs show that they were superbly healthy.

Therefore, first and foremost, the dog is a meat eater, its entire anatomy being adapted for a meat diet, from the teeth fashioned for tearing and crushing, the powerful jawbones and muscles, the small, very muscular stomach, the short intestines (to avoid putrefaction of flesh foods) and, above all, the very powerful digestive juices peculiar to the carnivorous animals – the digestive juices that can dissolve even lumps of bone. In health, the dog's juices, both of mouth and stomach, are strongly antiseptic, and thus 'high' meat and even flesh from diseased animals – food which would kill a human being in a day – can be eaten without harmful effects. But meat of an unnatural (very inflamed) colour should be avoided. It generally denotes previous high fever of the animal; dogs usually reject it.

The digestive capacity of the dog is very small when compared, for instance, with that of a goat – an animal of a size similar to some of the big-breed adults. The herbivorous animals – horses, cattle, etc – have enormous capacity for food and can consume many pounds of grain and herbage in a short space of time; whereas the dog, with its small stomach, has room for only very limited quantities of food. Consequently, the general feeding rule for dogs is small amounts of highly concentrated foods, of which raw meat is one of the foremost. Raw meat, fed in lumps, exercises to full capacity both the muscular stomach and the intestines, also the digestive juices, and, of course, utilizes the special teeth and jaw formation. If other food is substituted there is deterioration of the carnivorous organs of digestion. In view of all this, it is understandable that raw meat should form 75 per cent of the diet of every carnivorous animal.

On the subject of meat feeding, Shikari Man Mahipal Sinha, the chief hunter to the Maharajah of Namli, Central India, sent me an interesting letter. He fully agreed with my findings that a basically flesh diet is the only healthful one for all carnivorous animals, and his hunting hounds were all flesh fed. Only during the very hot seasons it became inadvisable to feed flesh, and the hounds were kept on a light diet of cooked whole-grain cereals, milk products, and similar food. The above findings are quite acceptable to me; I understand well that in countries of extreme climate, where dogs are employed in strenuous work, there are periods of heavy feeding (flesh diet) followed by long intervals of rest, when the dogs are kept on a semi-fasting diet. The Namli hunting hounds are kept on a light cereal diet, while, for instance, the Arctic sleigh dogs receive little food at all during the summer season. When they are retired from work and are turned loose they have to exist mainly on a diet of raw fish, much of which they must secure for themselves.

Meat is a highly concentrated food; for when the herbivorous animal is in good health its flesh should be made up of the important and highly nutritive vegetable foods on which it has nourished itself: green herbage, whole-grain cereals, sweet brook and spring waters, root vegetables, and silage (such foods are given in Natural Rearing of cattle, as opposed to the artificial cattle cake, acid-treated straw – even sawdust! – which produce sickly, unhealthy, overfat flesh). Raw flesh contains the cellulose of vegetable foods (which the dog can digest only with difficulty and in very limited quantities in the raw state) turned into protein by herbivorous digestion and now available as muscle, and easily assimilable by the dog. Such meat food has a fair vitamin and mineral content and is absolutely natural food for the dog, just as, to a similar extent, it is unnatural for the human being, to whom flesh food, because of its putrefactive nature, in combination with the human's non-carnivorous bodily structure (the lengthy digestive system), causes an excess of urine with consequential hardening of the human arteries and ligaments, leading to the unnatural onset of early senility. Flesh-eating animals void what they eat in approximately eight hours whereas human beings require, generally, forty-eight hours and have thirty feet of intestines to pass all food eaten. But there is no space here for reference to the vast subject of human diet. I must refer breeders to the excellent books on the subject by my friend Professor Dr Edmond Szekely (published by Keats Publishing Inc, New Canaan, USA, under the title *Three by Szekel*). But I should like to say that since human beings (fortunately) are unable to eat meat in its raw state, and therefore must cook all flesh foods, they thereby are losing most of the life-giving properties of that food; for cooking kills both vitamin content and those very valuable and as yet immeasurable cosmic forces, which collect in the flesh of herbivorous animals from the vegetable diet consumed.

Today there is little choice from the town butchers or general markets. The goat flesh and the sheep flesh on which the stalwart hunting hounds of the East are raised, and which are the type of flesh best suited to an animal of the dog's build, are rarely available. The toy breeds would thrive better on a diet of rabbit flesh or of poultry. I would suggest breeders make good use of such flesh foods as the following: breast of mutton (the small bones can also be fed, and are readily digestible by any dog in normal health, i.e. with strong, muscular intestines); sheep heads, including the very

7

nutritious eyes and brain (there is little risk of infection from the parasites that sometimes inhabit the brains of sheep; the good done by such foods offsets any slight risk there may be, since in any case a healthy animal is generally immune to the internal development of any parasite – worm or bacteria); ox cheeks, a readily digestible part of the carcass and rich in minerals (sheep heads and ox cheeks can be fed on the bone – the dog will readily tear off all the flesh); and paunches of all animals (the raw, uncleaned paunches of healthy grass-fed animals can be fed with much benefit to all breeds of dog). I learned this from a gypsy in the Forest of Dean: this man had bred many famous greyhounds, and he told me that such fare was the finest of natural food tonics. I have fed as he recommended, with great benefit to my dogs.

Needless to say, all the flesh foods given above are to be fed in their raw state only; no cooking of flesh foods can ever be tolerated in Natural Rearing (or NR). Guts of rabbits and hares can also be utilized. Rabbit guts can cause tapeworm, but the tapeworm is short-lived in the truly healthy dog; and in any case an orthodox diet of cooked foods is a far greater cause of long-duration tapeworm. Lewis Godfrey, of the Don Kennels, Hastings, Michigan, USA, writes very sensibly of the feeding of entrails to his borzois. He feeds all types: beef, chicken, fish. He emphasizes the richness of the fat which coats them, and states that most borzois lack fat in the diet. Lack of raw fat is indeed true of the orthodox diet of most breeds. However, only limited amounts should be given; for an average size dog, about one and a half dessertspoons per meal, several times a week. In the biblical dietary laws of Moses, fat is forbidden food for the Israelites. But it does contain that valuable vitamin, A.

Finally, how meat should be fed; the foremost law has just been given: *always* raw. Many veterinary surgeons – dominated by Pasteur's unnatural and faulty *germ theory of disease* –

advise the sterilizing, by cooking, of all meat fed to the dog. This was also the official ruling at the British Government dog-training centres (for war dogs), where the consequent health record of many dogs was unsatisfactory (much loss of young stock from disease, especially distemper, in spite of the distemper vaccination having been rigidly enforced). The main reason why dog owners cook meat is the sheer superstition that such food is made more safe. The theory is as outworn as that of Lister, who poured his ill-famed carbolic-acid disinfectants on to raw wounds in order to kill the 'disease' germs, and who thereby killed off all the beneficial bacteria which are responsible for tissue healing, and who consequently retarded (sometimes totally so) the healing of most wounds upon which his unnatural treatment was practised.

Destructive measures of any sort will never prove beneficial to life, and the feeding of meat or milk destroyed by being submitted to the forces of heat will only bring positive health degeneration, for nobody can know true health when fed on dead matter; and all cooked foods – with the exception of the naturally tough grains of cereals, which are well used to exposure to the burning heat of the sun's rays in their natural ripening and therefore to some extent resist the destructive forces of fire cooking – are unnatural, spoiled substances.

The cooking of meat is more mischievous in its results than the mere killing of the life forces which are present in all organic substances. Cooking semi-digests – artificially – the substance so treated; and in this unnatural breaking-down of the meat tissues, the rightful work of the stomach, intestines, and digestive juices having already been undertaken before the food is fed to the dog, these organs are left improperly exercised; and when this procedure is repeated day after day, it is understandable – it is indeed a law of Nature – they will soften and atrophy, so that in time they will be unable to cope with their natural work. Further, the delicate taste buds of the mouth will have become what in medical parlance is known as 'depraved', due to an aberration from natural diet; the high-tasting properties of cooked flesh will cause dogs to reject their normal diet of raw flesh for the palate-excitant one of cooked food. Appetite and food preferences, as with man, are no guide to the suitability of foods for the domestic dog. For, resulting from the feeding of unnatural foods for many generations, diet tastes can become perverted.

Now, thousands of dogs – in fact, when pets are taken into the counting, the majority of dogs – are fed habitually on a cooked-foods diet: many are deprived altogether of meat foods; and dogs so fed survive. It is true they are hosts for a multitude of worms, they have unpleasant body smells, have bad breath, and age rapidly; 70 per cent of them have disordered kidneys by their seventh year, also failing eyesight and hearing; their teeth are so filthy with a brown 'fur' deposit that they have to be scraped regularly by a veterinary surgeon. But they survive. How very different is the effect of such diet upon an animal whose ancestors have been reared on a strict raw-foods diet for many generations, and who has been weaned and reared through half of its puppyhood period on the selfsame diet, when it is suddenly placed on foods which are entirely foreign to its system – filthy foods. The harmful effect upon the body, including the nervous system, can well be imagined and understood. Therefore, when you strictly Nature Rear any stock, take precautions that those who acquire your animals will continue with the same health diet. I personally, as well as many other breeders, can promptly tell from examination of the teeth, limbs, and eyes whether or not an animal is being Naturally Reared, and we are seldom mistaken. As many breeders have told me: 'Nature Reared stock look so different! They are so vitally alive!' When one meets them in the show ring, the naturally reared stock make the other stock look stiff and aged; it is no wonder that at the present time so many of the c.c. winners at dog shows are NR stock.

One of the worst faults of cooked flesh and most other cooked foods, especially milk – cooking having changed the nature of the substance – is the after effect when kept for any length of time. This is entirely different from the natural. Raw flesh, when kept for many days, especially during warm weather, becomes 'high' or 'gamey'; it acquires a strong smell; sometimes, also, a grey mould forms; internally, it becomes very tender. It can be fed to any animal with perfect safety, it being quite natural for the dog to partake of flesh in such a state. Indeed, the digging-up and eating of long-buried flesh is one of the delights of the truly healthy dog whose natural instincts have not been spoiled by a cooked-foods diet, for it must always be remembered that *the dog is a natural scavenger* just as much as he is a killer. Very different is cooked meat after storing for many days. This meat turns green in hue and becomes sweaty. To feed 'high' cooked meat is to feed true poison in every sense of the word.

Mr J. Fairfax-Blakeborough, whose always interesting articles, in *Dog World* (of England) and elsewhere, which reveal him as being a true student and lover of Nature, upholds my persistent writings on the essential feeding of flesh foods in their raw state. He also makes mention of the old-time greyhound breeders' preference for mutton, this food having always been my own preference for all dogs other than the very big breeds, who can fare quite well on the coarser horse or cow flesh. To quote from Mr Fairfax-Blakeborough in *Dog World*:

A friend of mine who has somehow managed to keep a considerable number of terriers, hounds and other dogs during the war years, argues in favour of raw-meat feeding. If dogs find a buried sheep they dig it up and eat it, and seem to relish and thrive on such carrion, so that I am not at all sure that this is not *getting very near to Nature, upon which man can rarely improve.* [My italics.] Dining the other evening with Mr D.W.E. Brock, who had just taken over the amalgamated Cumberland packs, he told me that he had found feeding raw flesh produced the hardiest and fittest hounds, that he does not think kennels will ever go back to oatmeal on the same scale, and although he has had on occasion to boil flesh to prevent it from becoming tainted, he has often fed hounds when it was 'not all that it should be' without any ill results. [If kennel owners would acquire the habit of digging deep pits among the roots of a shady tree, and placing the meat therein, all the problems of flesh becoming tainted would be overcome, as buried meat 'ripens', it does not taint – J. de B.L.] ... Then followed an interesting discussion whether such carcasses could not well be used in view of the natural habits of the canine species, which preferred meat which had been buried for some time, and which seemed to prove by subsequent coat and condition that it suited them.

I often feel when thinking back on my canine work, that if I am able to instil two reforms into the canine world: the fasting of all dogs in sickness, and the strict feeding of only raw flesh – never cooked meat in any form – then my years of canine work will not have been wasted.

The problem of keeping raw meat safe from the ravaging attacks of blowflies during the spring and summer months is not an easy one, especially when large quantities are in use and the kennels are situated a considerable distance from a meat supplier. That is one of the reasons why kennels of few inmates are advocated in preference to over-populated ones.

Fifteen Afghan hounds (including the puppies) was the largest number of dogs that I ever kept at one time, and that number was too many. I was able to have raw meat available for them always, including the hottest months of summer, for I used the ancient Eastern way of burying the meat in the ground in a shady place.

BURIED MEAT

The meat must be free from all fly eggs, for otherwise these will hatch out, even after deep burial, and will spoil the meat. If fly-blown, *all* the eggs must be scraped off carefully and the cleansed meat then patted over with a swab of cotton dipped in vinegar. These eggs are seen in patches on the meat, a crowd of minute, elongated, white specks.

If the eggs have actually hatched out into maggots, no need to throw the meat away. It can be cleansed of the maggots by vigorous sluicing down with water; then rub the meat briskly with vinegar and finally pat in a little salt. Fly maggots should not, of course, be eaten by dogs because the bluebottle or blowfly, which lays the eggs on meat, specially seeks out rotting flesh and may well carry disease from its feet and body touch on meat, or through its maggots.

The pit dug should be a deep one, for sufficient coolness during hot weather, and the floor should be lined with tree branches or slabs of stone; tree branches or stone slabs should also be placed over the meat before replacing the soil. These will protect the meat against over-soiling, not that a little soil matters when it is clean. This burying method keeps the meat well and also 'ripens' it. A gypsy told me how his people ripen apples (wild crab apples) by digging pits in the ground, lining the pits with straw, and placing the apples therein. Apples can be kept for months that way.

The pit area should be in tree shade preferably, and must be marked with a stout stick, otherwise it may be difficult to find. An uncorked bottle half filled with turpentine, placed on the buried meat area, gives a strong smell and helps in keeping insects from finding the buried meat. This may read like a lot of trouble, but far less trouble than washing greasy food dishes and pans, resultant from cooked-meat feeding, and nursing diseased animals also resultant from such feeding.

Stonehenge, the great British canine writer of ancient times, advocated giving raw flesh a coat of whitewash and hanging it in the shade of a tree in order to preserve it. He stated that flesh so treated would keep edible for a month or more.

Flesh may be kept for a long time even in summer, by brushing it over with a quick-lime wash, or dusting it with the powder, and then hanging it up in trees with thick foliage. In this way I have kept the shank ends of legs and shoulders good for six weeks in the height of summer and in the winter for three months.

Small amounts of meat can be placed in brown paper bags or cotton flour bags, the necks tied with string to prevent fly penetration, and hung from a wire coat hanger on a shady tree branch. The wire hook of the hanger will usually deter ants, but if they should defy this, a piece of cloth must be soaked in paraffin daily and wound around the hook base of the hanger; ants will not walk over paraffin. Vinegar can be used on such meat as a mild preservative, using two table-spoons to one cup of water. Then wrap the meat around with big green leaves, or meat can be salted.

And, after all, there is always refrigeration! If this is on low freezing, little harm will be done to the health properties of the meat. But hard freezing is as destructive as cooking to the health of the meat and to those who consume it. Therefore never put meat in the freezer. Frozen (iced) food should be used with great caution as it causes ulceration of the digestive tract. I have noted the care peasants take to prevent their animals from eating roots and other crops touched by frost. Refrigerated meat must be thawed out and, if necessary, well scalded with hot water. Make sure the thawing is complete before giving it to the dog. I repeat, iced meat is dangerous.

In the wild, hair and underskin are part of a natural flesh diet and supply essential roughage to exercise the strong muscles of the digestive tract, acting also as a mild laxative. Since in our time the tanner claims animal hides, a little bran should be used instead. Bran supplies roughage and also vitamin B. It has little food value, but it is of a protein nature, although a cereal product. Merely sprinkle a small quantity of bran over the meat feed for each dog; bran ration for an average dog is about one tablespoon. When bran is unobtainable, a little flaked oats can be used. Oats also are roughage and protein rich. A small sprinkle will not break the cereal-and-protein-separation rule. When possible, feed meat on the bone in order to encourage the use of the natural canine tearing action. Many of my hounds have swallowed rabbits whole, their strong digestive organs being well able to dissolve and digest the prey, including hair and bones.

Ground-up (minced) meat is especially bad for health as it deprives the dog of jaw and intestinal exercise. Also it often contains too much fat and is harmful, therefore, to health of liver and arteries.

Animals in the wild, after tearing off some outer skin and flesh of their victims, unfailingly show a preference for certain organs of the body: first the intestines, then the eyes. The intestines supply a good source of semi-digested starch and green herbage in the vegetable-eating animals on which the canine races prey usually. (The subject of starch will be fully dealt with subsequently.) The other chosen organs are the eyes, which animals gouge out with great eagerness. (Sea-gulls, which are partly carnivorous, always greedily seek the eyes of drowned bodies, animal or human.) It is no doubt some minerals salts which attract the carnivorous animals, phosphorus and iodine normally being present in the eye tissue. Dr Weston A. Price, writing in a dental journal concerning the Indian tribes of northern Canada, states: '. . . they know that the tissues forming the back part of the eye are good for food. Science has recently demonstrated that the retina of the eyes is one of the rich sources of vitamin A.' The teeth are never acceptable, even as roughage, unless the animal is swallowed whole in the case of rabbits and other lesser prey on which the carnivores feed; they are then expel-led in the faeces.

RABBITS AND POULTRY Rabbits and hares are among the best and most natural sources of protein for the dog. Their sharp-splintering bones can be dangerous, especially when cooked. But when the rabbit is eaten by the dog in its natural form – whole, including hair, etc – the hairy skin prevents any danger from bones splintering and puncturing the stomach or intestines.

That loathsome man-caused rabbit disease, myxomatosis, so far has not been found harmful to dogs although some hares have died from myxomatosis. If any dogs should get the disease they should be treated as described for Distemper and Hard Pad.

It must be added that, in order to feed rabbits and poultry raw, they should be used fresh, when the flesh is still warm. The flesh of such animals stiffens when cold and becomes rather indigestible.

Therefore, when feeding long-killed shop-bought rabbits, it is advisable to dip the flesh in hot – just off the boil – water and keep submerged for two to three minutes. This will restore the natural elasticity of the flesh without destructive cooking. Some bran or oat flakes should be added as roughage substitute for hair or feathers and to prevent bone-piercing danger.

The same treatment applies to poultry, the flesh needing some quick softening in a little hot water.

LIVER The dog's natural craving for this organ of the animal body is explained by its high vitamin content and the rich source of natural minerals found in this organ. Liver has long been an accredited cure for anaemia in human beings, but there is a unique acid present in liver, and this is solely derived from the green 'blood' of leaves; indeed, the acid was named folic acid, from *folia* – leaf. Common sense would indicate that, in the case of human beings who are well able to assimilate vegetable matter, it would be far more practical to obtain the leaf acid from its source, raw green salads, than indirectly through the liver organ of any animal!

Just as animals seek out the eyes and intestines of their prey, they also seek the liver and the adrenal glands. Indeed, an animal which has not had its natural instincts thwarted and undermined has a very definite plan of action when partaking of the body of its prey. The liver is frequently a very unhealthy organ in an unclean animal, however, as it is the great biochemist of the body, handling many toxic substances, and therefore often overworked. It is one of the first organs to become diseased when the health of the body declines. It can become the storeplace for all manner of body impurities and toxins. In the sheep it can be infected with fluke, a dangerous parasite. Therefore, only feed liver when it is known beyond all doubt that it comes from a healthy animal. Even so, liver is a common cause of diarrhoea in dogs and cats so feed sparingly, not more than twice a week. It is a definite fact that my Afghan hounds refuse most internal organs of poultry and the bigger meat animals, and they always refuse liver and kidneys. This refusal seems to be some inherited tribal law.

TRIPE AND THROAT These are suitable foods when raw, fresh, and tender. The flesh has to be cut up in quite small pieces. Once frozen or cooked, it becomes indigestible.

CANNED MEAT This is an unnatural food and causes over-eating and bloating. Nature never taught the dog either to cook or to use a can-opener! It is understandable that an amount of chemical preservative is nearly always utilized to keep such food from souring. The food is 'dead' matter in every sense of the word. The spices and other flavouring materials with which it is generally mixed induce artificial hunger in the dog to which it is fed, and this may damage the stomach lining and the normal balance of the digestive juices. How can any thinking person expect to keep an animal really healthy on preserved food from a tin or bottle? The popularity of such food, supported by large-scale and clever advertising, in my opinion is one reason for the extraordinary increase and variety in canine disease today, when it has become quite usual to feed dogs largely on such totally unnatural fare. Canned meat usually produces over-copious faeces of bad odour. This causes a disgraceful situation on paths and roadways worldwide and when deposited on fields the earth is soured.

A warning should be given that in the rampant commercialism of modern times, cheapness of ingredients is too often the basic consideration and necessity. Like the title of a once-popular song, 'Anything goes', which means that such things as dried blood are used – blood scraped from the floors of the world's slaughter-houses, charged with harmful adrenalin which floods the bloodstream of terrified animals at slaughter time. Massive fish waste resulting from the death of shoals of fish is also used.

BONES   When fed raw, they are the canine and feline toothbrush. Through exercise, they also improve jaw structure and strength and promote the length of the jaw. I have always had exceptional foreface on my Afghan hounds, and I know that jaw exercise (plus the feeding of powdered seaweed) has been the reason for this. Bones also exercise the salivary glands. Soft bones are best for regular use, or flat bones such as ribs, because the hard (marrow-filled) ones are apt to wear down the teeth unduly. Bones which splinter and bones small enough for the dog to swallow whole, as well as cooked poultry and sharp fish bones, should be avoided. They can puncture the intestines and cause death. Sheep heads, sliced in half, are good and can be fed frequently with the flesh in, for the dog to pick clean. An old-fashioned food for foxhounds is quickly obtained by boiling a whole sheep with the wool on it and pouring the resultant stock, when tepid, over oatmeal cereal. Personally I do not feed soup of any kind to my dogs or cats as this dirties the stomach and intestinal tract, but for those who wish to do so, the foxhound kennel's way is useful. The brains' content of sheep heads is very rich in minerals, and dogs will eat it raw. A heavy shin bone sawn up by the butcher into manageable proportions is the best bone food for dogs. Any marrow which the dog cannot reach can be forked out and mixed with the meat later. Bones should be fed after meals only, not given on an empty stomach when they could puncture an intestine or create intestinal gas. But do remember that meat fed *without* bones is unnatural.

Do not leave bones lying around in dog runs to invite flies and rodents.

CHICKEN LEGS   Fed raw, provide a most excellent soft bony food very rich in calcium and much enjoyed by all dogs. The nails should be cut off and discarded, and the legs well washed. They should be lightly crushed for toy breeds to enable them to be eaten more easily.

FISH

Fish is not a recommended canine food. It is too watery and bloodless for the carnivores. However, some breeds of dogs, especially the Portuguese water spaniels who catch fish for themselves, and some species of Arctic dogs, get almost a mono-diet of fish and flourish on such diet. But they will be obtaining their fish sea- or river-fresh and therefore the flesh is supple and easily digested. The strong, healthy natives of many islands of the South Seas spear and eat raw, sea-fresh fish. Fish many hours old must be treated the same way as advised for rabbits and poultry, that is, scalded well with hot water to remove the unnatural stiffening of the flesh. On my travels I have quite often seen cats catching fish in shallow pools, scooping them out with their paws and eating them whole – raw, of course.

Mackerel and herring are the best fish for canine diet, being extra rich in fats (often lacking in canine diet), nerve vitamin B, and vital minerals. The innards should always be fed, only the heads discarded. A sprinkle of flaked oats is healthful with such rich fish. It can be fed once or twice a week as a change from raw meat. Canned tuna fish is nutritious; its only preservatives are salt and oil, though modern tuna has become suspect because of harmful chemicals found in it from factory wastes discharged into the world's seas.

Lightly steamed white fish, such as cod, plaice, etc, is the ideal 'first' protein for an invalid diet, to be followed by raw meat (see Internal Cleansing Diet, p. 139).

GENERAL FEEDING (CEREALS)

Cereal feeding is of far less importance than meat feeding, but it is important enough, for it is on cereals that carnivorous life relies for most of the all-essential minerals as well as the majority of vitamins, including the vital fertility vitamin E, present in the germ of cereals, especially in wheat and maize.

The immense feeding value in cereals can be understood when one stops to think upon the magnificent health of a bull or stallion, raised on a vegetable diet. Dog owners who feed only meat and exclude cereals altogether are making a dietary error, and animals so fed cannot possibly enjoy total health; their diet being one-sided will likewise give one-sided health. Equally bad is the feeding of popular white-flour cereals, for the food value of such is almost nil: all the essential minerals, vitamins, and cosmic forces which account for the dog's need for cereals are totally lacking in white flour, which merely forms a gluey paste in the stomach, the cause of the prevalent canine gastric disorders and general deficiency diseases, including rickets. It should be remembered that the dog always obtained some semi-digested cereals in his diet. His first action in killing his prey was – and still is – to rip open the abdomen and devour the grains and vegetable matter contained in the intestines of the usually herbivorous prey. So dogs would also obtain some barks of trees from the intestines of rabbits or goats, excellent food for dogs.

In selecting a balanced diet for dogs one should always remember to include the sort of foods which the prey – rabbit, goat, etc – eat, and which the killer dog would get from the intestines of the prey.

Such grains, vegetables, herbs and barks obtained in that way would be semi-digested by the prey before its death. As the vegetable-eating animals chew and salivate, much digestion takes place in the mouth as well as in the intestines; they do not bolt food whole as do the carnivores. Therefore, it is understandable that, unlike flesh food, cereal grains fresh from the plant itself cannot be digested by the dog, such food generally passing through the intestines of the dog almost untouched. (It must be mentioned that during the modern worldwide myxomatosis plague, artificially spread by man among the rabbit population, the fox was found to be robbing the wheat when starved of its largely rabbit diet. Intestines of slain foxes were filled with wheat and oats direct from the plants, and the animals avoided starvation that way. This shows that, when compelled, carnivores can eat raw cereals.)

Some preparation of cereals is required for dogs, and the best method is flaking of the cereal by passing it through heated rollers, as is done in the flour mills. (Wheat needs different treatment, and should be ground finely and lightly cooked in order to render it digestible.) Flaked cereals should be soaked overnight in cold vegetable stock, plain cold milk, or buttermilk. I do want to emphasize that flaked cereals are the most economical and healthful ways of feeding cereals to dogs and cats.

For ages Border collies on English farms shared the sacks of flaked maize with the farm animals, the maize merely soaked in whey for the dogs. But I have pioneered a full range of flaked cereals for dogs, and benefits to health have been remarkable. Only half the amount of flaked cereals is needed compared with fully cooked bread or biscuit food. *Do remember this teaching* and try your dogs and cats on natural, flaked cereals, but take care what you buy because nowadays many flaked cereals are, for commercial purposes 'roasted' further after flaking. This gives more commercial protection against moths and weevils, which like to feed on healthful, flaked cereals and are not interested in eating the more lifeless, extra-cooked cereals and bread and biscuits.

Personally, I do not use meat or fish stock for my dogs as it is apt to sour the cereals and likewise sour the intestines. Another reason why I oppose the use of meat or fish stock is that such are commonly used in laboratories as media for the cultivation of disease bacteria.

Young corn (maize) can be fed raw from the fields when the cobs are young and milky. Merely grate the grains (kernels) finely with a vegetable-shredder, then mix with a little vegetable oil and milk and add a pinch of salt. I feed this often to my Afghan hounds and to my children. One can keep corn fresh after gathering or buying it by standing the whole cobs, stalks down, in a basin of water.

Dog owners can bake their own *wholewheat* dog cakes (soft), using the speedy way of the Bedouin Arabs. Merely mix several pounds of slightly warmed wholewheat flour, using warm water or buttermilk, honey and molasses (two tablespoons), salt (two teaspoons), added to every quart of water used. Leave in a warm place to rise a little (without yeast). After fifteen minutes, make a hole in the centre of the dough and pour in two dessertspoons of olive oil (or corn oil) to every two pounds of wholewheat flour used. Leave to rise a further thirty minutes, then sprinkle with a little dry flour and form into small flat cakes. Bake on oiled trays in a hot oven for approximately forty minutes. The aim is quick baking to prevent destruction of the vital wheat germ. Solid 'Arabian' cakes result, excellent for teeth and jaw development. My children also flourished on such fare. I do not use yeast often despite the praise given to it by the medical profession; it is an active ferment and can convey the fermentation to the stomach and other organs, causing much internal upset. Professor Edmond Szekeley, author of many books on natural diet and a world-famed authority on diet, warns against the use of yeast. The Bedouins also make *petah*. The flour is then almost raw; unleavened, it is merely cooked a few minutes on hot metal plates.

When in southern Spain I learned to make *toasted* flour, using wholewheat or wholemaize (corn) flour. When made, it is served semi-liquid with cold, raw milk, or made into small balls to eat raw, using tepid water, olive oil, and salt. To toast flour, place in an iron frying-pan ¼lb flour, spread out well by shaking, then place the pan containing the dry flour over a low flame (preferably using an asbestos mat beneath the pan, but not essential). With the blade of a knife, constantly lift the flour and turn it over, until all deepens into a pale gold (or dark gold, if yellow corn flour is used). The toasting usually takes around five minutes. Shake the pan frequently. When toasted, allow the flour to cool; then store in tins. A hot oven can also be used for toasting, after the heat has been turned off. In this method, shake and mix the flour well several times to prevent burning. The famed greyhounds of Seville and Cordoba are given *harina tostada* – and flourish on it.

There is also the *migas* of the Spanish and Portuguese peasants, which I learned to make for my children and dogs while in those lands. Into a pan of slightly salted cold water (approximately a quart), toss six 'teeth' cloves of raw garlic and a few sprigs of thyme, sage, or rosemary, one tablespoon olive or corn oil. Then stir in spoonfuls of wholewheat or maize flour, an approximate ½lb of flour to a quart of water. Cook slowly and stir well throughout the cooking, which takes approximately fifteen minutes. Then, when thickened, turn heat very low, place lid on pan, and cook slowly for two or three minutes. When cold, cut into slices and serve. It can be buttered for extra good taste. Chopped herbs such as chives, mint, parsley, etc, can be added when cold. In sunny climates it is helpful to soak the flour in warm water for several hours, placed out in the full sunlight; it will then cook more easily.

OATS   Flaked, as sold in packets, they are a vital canine food. Being a very good source of iron, they also cleanse the intestines of impurities. They are a proved vital food for stud dogs and brood bitches. It is on oatmeal porridge that the famous collie dogs of Scotland and other hill regions of Great Britain have been reared. These dogs are known for their stamina and resistance to cold and damp. The Border collie is one of the few natural domestic breeds still unspoiled by man, and its health record is enviable compared to that of most domestic breeds ill-reared for generations on unnatural foods.

Packet oat flakes are already pre-cooked during the flaking. Do not cook further, merely soak overnight in cold milk, or cold watered milk or cold vegetables, not meat, soup (nettles and shredded carrot are excellent for this, also potato skins and pea-pods left over from the household kitchen). Add a little salt. 'Milk of oats' is an excellent invalid drink. Merely pour one quart of hot (not boiling) water over a large handful of flaked oats. Allow to stand overnight. Then strain off the liquid 'milk' by pressing this all out from the oats. Reheat to tepid only, then stir in a pinch of salt and one dessertspoon of honey or of maple syrup.

BARLEY   This is a great aid in dog rearing because of its medicinal properties apart from its considerable food value. It is rich in the antacid magnesium, and is indeed the most alkaline of the cereals. It is an excellent blood cleanser and blood cooler during the hot weather. The Arabs choose barley as the principal cereal for their fine Arabian horses and greyhounds (salukis).

The soothing property of barley flour makes it of value also for external use, and a poultice of barley flour was once a well-known remedy in old English and French homes for treatment of skin ailments. Barley is also a good kidney remedy, and drinks of barley water should be given daily in kidney diseases, and in ailments of the bladder.

RYE This is an excellent cereal as a change, but the rye used must be whole grain. In its outer coat it contains fluorine, responsible for the formation of good tooth enamel and strong nails. Being low in carbohydrate and fat content, it is a good food for overweight dogs. It is also good for miniature toy breeds, as it keeps them tiny. It is best fed as rye 'wafers', obtainable in packets from food stores.

CORN (maize) This wonderful cereal, worshipped by the ancient Red Indians and Mexicans, is the only cereal able to sustain life for many months as a sole food. It is usually fed to the dog pre-cooked and flaked. It is then apt to be overeaten and heats the blood unduly. One handful of flaked maize is sufficient daily ration for an average size adult dog. The young cobs can be fed raw, merely grated on a vegetable shredder and mixed with milk. The centre core, to which the kernels were attached, is discarded. This cereal, being sun-charged, is a vital one for fertility, being an excellent glandular tonic. It is one of the supreme foods for growing beautiful and abundant hair and strong teeth.

It is said that two foods do not lose their vitamins when canned: corn and pineapple. Dogs and cats much enjoy canned sweet-corn, as a change from the fresh and during those months when fresh corn is not in season. Cream-style corn is the best, but if the whole kernel is given, then the kernels should be mashed small for digestibility. Corn is my favourite of the cereals, a liking shared by my dogs. As for cats, I have seen them go quite crazy with pleasure when they get the strong scent from a newly opened can of corn. I do not uphold canned food, but a treat of corn does good now and then – and how far better than a can of meat, which I totally avoid!

Corn *oil* is valuable; several teaspoons can be added to the mixed cereal feed for an average size dog. Avoid degerminated corn flours. The 'silk' of corn, the tangle of threads found on the outer cobs, provides an excellent remedy for all kidney ailments. It is fed uncooked, finely minced, or made into a tea. Two teaspoons of silk daily, for an average size dog.

After many years of trying, I was able in the 1960s to supply for followers of Natural Rearing a complete food of the four cereals – oats, barley, rye and corn – blended with sea-salt, dried carrots and herbs. Sold as Natural Rearing flakes, the food has enjoyed long success and now has many imitations. (Address, p. 320.)

RICE   Dogs enjoy an occasional meal of rice, especially when it is enriched with vegetable oils, such as olive or corn, added when the rice is cold, and a raw egg. The natural brown rice from grocers and health foods shops is best. This cereal, *Oryza sativa*, when it is natural 'native' rice, is famous for its health properties, including its ability to cure dysentery. The properties are thiamine, niacin and iron, and they are lost during the polishing of rice from its natural brown form into unnatural white. If only white rice is obtainable, then add one tablespoon of wheat bran per cupful of rice to restore some vitamin content and roughage. Nowadays, rice flakes are obtainable.

LINSEED   This is a valuable winter tonic when fed in small quantities along with the other cereal foods. Linseed is rich in minerals, and its valuable oil is very fattening and is a wonderful hair and nerve tonic when used internally – or externally as a hair stimulant and general massage aid. But linseed cake should be avoided, as it is merely the compressed residue of the seed after the valuable oil has been removed by crushing. Linseed must be prepared carefully, for otherwise, owing to its very tough outer coat, it remains entirely inedible and contains a harmful acid. The seed should be soaked in much water for twenty-four hours. Throw away that water. Next day cook slowly for about thirty minutes, stirring repeatedly in order to prevent its adhering to the pan sides and burning. The fluid obtained during the cooking should not be thrown out, for it possesses valuable mineral salts and some oil. It should be used as a base for other soup, reboiling it along with vegetable wastes, leaves, onion and potato skins, etc. Do not add meat.

Linseed can also be prepared, soaked raw, in the same way as bean sprouts.

PULSES: BEANS, PEAS, LENTILS, FENUGREEK, SESAME

These foods, rich in nitrates and fats, are much used in Spain, Mexico and the Central Americas for cattle dogs, which do well on them. At least such food is whole and has not had germ and outer layers removed in processing, as with most cereals.

All should be soaked overnight in cold water, with a pinch of bicarbonate of soda added to reduce the need for lengthy cooking. To cook, place in boiling water and cook rapidly in as little water as possible until soft enough to be digestible. Flavour with a little salt and add some oil when cold. A small quantity of apple or citrus vinegar, one teaspoon to every one and a half pints of water in which the beans are cooked, lessens the health-destructive cooking time. The Arabian *hilbeh* – fenugreek seed – merely soak, without soda, and feed raw, one tablespoon per dog; very nutritious. Fenugreek is of the legumes family, botanical name *Trigonella foenum-graecum*. It can be prepared, sprouted, as with linseed.

SPROUTED FOODS   Sprouted pulses (beans, etc) are a popular modern health food for human use. Sprouted grains and pulses can be prepared at home, or bought ready sprouted from supermarkets and health stores. Soak grains or pulses until they sprout well. They can then be crushed well and eaten raw. They give much vitality and vitamins. Remember when putting them to sprout that they should be rinsed morning and night.

SOYA BEANS   In modern times they have become quite popular as a dog food, but as they are both indigestible and fermentative, I avoid them. The fact that soya cannot be fed raw is a black mark against its value. I find it a trouble-maker.

SESAME (*Sesamum indicum*)   This is the oil-rich seed of an Eastern plant. The crushed seeds make a thick, creamy, oily substance called *tahina*. This is excellent for all dogs and much liked by them, and is easily digested. Add to milk. One dessertspoon of *tahina* three or four times weekly with the cereal feed (for an average size dog). The crushed seeds – lightly roasted and made into a paste by pouring over them liquid honey, forked into flat slabs, lightly cooked in a moderately hot oven and, when set, cut into squares – make an excellent sweetmeat for dogs, as 'treats' for good behaviour. I use sesame pieces to train my Afghan hounds, as a reward for returning when called, this breed being a very wayward one. They have a passion for sesame. Sesame bars can be purchased in grocers' shops and kiosks throughout the Middle East where they are very popular and valued for health-giving qualities; also now available in health food shops worldwide.

ROOT VEGETABLES

TURNIPS, PARSNIPS, SWEET POTATOES (yams), JERUSALEM (tuber) ARTICHOKES   All are nutritious and rich in vitamins and minerals. They should be either baked in an oven or sliced for quick boiling in a little hot, salted water. They are best when fed mashed into grain cereals. Parsnips and turnips, boiled and spread on to linen cloths when hot, make excellent poultices for swollen limbs, boils, etc. I do not feed common potato; it is too watery for a canine food and also causes stomach gas and colic.

CARROTS   A root vegetable rich in vitamins and minerals (when properly grown by organic methods), they make an excellent supplement for the canine cereal feed and are blood cleansing and worm removing. Prepare as advised for the other root vegetables. Also feed a little raw, very finely grated. That way carrots are likely to expel worms. Carrots aid formation of good tooth enamel, and are a good eye tonic. Scrub carrots very well, sprinkle with salt, keep salted for several hours, then rinse very well. This preparation is a precaution against parasite flukes which can attack the liver and kill the host animal.

MILK FOODS AND HERBS

MILK   This will be dealt with in some detail in the section on puppy weaning and therefore will only receive brief mention now. For it must be understood that milk is not a natural food for the dog; the food is natural to human children, whose parents have for centuries kept cattle for the purpose of milk production, and whose anatomy is best suitable to a vegetable diet – milk *is* vegetable matter, in liquid form, as produced by the grass – and herb-eating cow or goat. But to the older puppy and to the older dog, milk is not a natural food, and when taken in excess it will form mucus deposits, which are frequently the root cause of many of the common canine ailments, especially worm infection. Milk should be reserved for the weaning of puppies and the early feeding of weaned stock, especially in the big breeds when much rapid growth must be fostered; for bitches suckling their young; and for treatment of sick or thin animals. The milk-honey diet for sick animals simply cannot be improved on, and for that reason alone, no person should attempt puppy rearing who is unable to ensure supplies of fresh raw milk at all times. Needless to say, just as it is essential to ensure that cereal foods are obtained from healthy grain, so likewise milk must be of high health standard, obtained from healthy cows or goats. Disease can be fed to puppies through unclean and unhealthy milk, just as it can through rodent-tainted grain. Care must always be taken to ensure that only healthy foods are fed to all animals on all occasions. I have usually kept my own goats when rearing many young puppies.

Avoid modern long-life milk. Its true name should be 'short-life'; it is a dead fluid and clogs the internal organs in the same way as that other long-life substance, margarine.

BUTTERMILK This excellent food is an acquired taste in dogs and they should be given it from early puppyhood. Similar to whole, sour 'clabbered' milk, it has worm-removing properties. It is also very blood cooling. It makes a perfect biscuit base, with wholewheat flour mixed purely with buttermilk instead of the plain water usually used in baking of biscuits.

The secret of making good clabbered milk – and therefore buttermilk – is to keep the milk aerated during the making. The milk should stand in a warm place, or in sunlight, and be topped with thin paper or cotton to keep out flies or dust. Do not sunheat above tepid. The standing milk should be stirred briskly with a fork, morning, midday, and night.

BUTTER This being an unnatural food, it should be used very sparingly, as it is apt to cause liver trouble in dogs and cats, despite their enjoyment of this food. It can be spread lightly on wholewheat or wholerye bread, and in this way helps to encourage appetite in poor eaters.

CHEESE Fresh white cheese or cottage cheese is a good food which most dogs, and some cats, enjoy. Solid yellow cheese is indigestible. If used it should be grated finely.

HERBS Most herbs play a very small part in canine diet, although a remarkably important part in canine medicine. The dog is no true vegetable eater, taking only what it gets from the contents of the intestines of the prey which it kills, and in very limited amounts direct from various grasses, berries, and mosses, which it seeks out for itself. Many dogs have completely lost their natural instincts for the seeking-out of herbs; only for that admirable, intestinal cleansing herb, couch grass (*Agropyrum repens*), do dogs seem to have retained their herb-eating instinct, and even this instinct is often thwarted by their owners, who drag their dogs away from the grass because they do not like its making their dogs vomit up bile, which is the sole purpose, apart from its laxative properties, for which the dog eats couch grass! Modern veterinary surgeons have also been known to advise clients to keep their dogs away from couch grass because it will cause vomiting and loose bowels. Yet this grass is so important for maintaining health in dogs and cats that, if not available as a wild plant, roots should be procured and planted where dogs and cats can utilize them.

FRUITS

The dog and even the cat will eat many varieties of fruits and berries with much pleasure. They do not have to obtain such foods only from intestines of prey; they can eat and digest fruits direct from bush or tree. The Bible tells us of the pleasure that the fox takes in eating grapes. My Afghan hounds also enjoy grapes and will lap up fresh grape juice. My Irish wolfhound bitch was a great eater of berries and she would find for me the places where the wild raspberries grew.

Lady Rose of Edinburgh told me of her currant bushes and how they were grazed avidly by her spaniels, and I used to see the lurcher dogs of the New Forest gypsies raiding the strawberry fields, eating up large quantities of the fruit.

In the Middle East the jackals are tiresome in the melon fields as they go from fruit to fruit taking a few bites and spoiling them. The passion that cats have for cucumbers is well known. It is believed they eat them as a worm preventative and remedy, small melons too.

NUTS

Nuts of all kinds are enjoyed by dogs. Many dogs will themselves crack open walnuts and hazel nuts and carefully extract the contents, discarding all the bad pieces. In the main, nuts should be crushed for the dogs (as they would get them in the intestines of their prey). Nuts provide natural oils and many vitamins and minerals. As a tonic for thin dogs and for special pups, I grind the nuts into powder using a small handmill, and mix the flour into milk.

GROUND NUTS (peanuts)   Although not a true nut, they are also suitable food for dogs. On Spanish farms I saw the cattle dogs raiding the fields for newly planted ground nuts which they ate in quantities. Pine kernels are also not true nuts, but excellent nourishment. Use in the same way as nuts. All are expensive food items, but far cheaper than buying vitamin pills, etc.

Peanut flour is a useful and cheap addition to canine and feline diet as it is rich in oils and minerals and, being of the legumes family, is rich in the important substance nitrate; the flour, added to cereals, is a great body builder. The nuts used to make the flour must be raw; if roasted they are very indigestible. As peanuts grow beneath the soil it is not usually a sprayed crop. The nuts soon turn rancid and ferment easily and are then dangerous, so it is best to grind fresh nuts – in the same way as other nuts – when needed: the process takes only a few minutes. Shelled almonds can also be made into highly nutritious flour. It is not necessary to blanch them of their skins because that loses minerals. The amount of peanut or almond flour to use is a dessertspoon a few days a week for the average size dog.

WATER

The bodies of humans and animals are approximately 70 per cent water, and the dog parts with a large amount of this daily via the lungs and urinary organs. Loss of urine is especially heavy after active exercise. Therefore, for health maintenance there must be a constant renewal of the water content of the body by regular intake of this highly important fluid. The dog, especially when sick, can exist for days and weeks solely on water, whereas in general he could not live for more than a limited number of days without intake of water, though there have been exceptions to this fact in the case of dogs lost down badger holes, old mines, trapped in bombed buildings, etc, which have survived for weeks even without water.

The water, which the dog replaces daily, must be pure and natural for total health. In the past, when purchasing Afghan hounds to establish my own Turkuman strain, one of my first considerations was the water supply of the kennel that I was visiting. I always sought stock from country kennels where there was good water. A famous race-horse breeder once told me that he would not consider land for his mares and foals where there was not a running stream of spring-fed water. He wanted strong bones for the legs of his race-horses, and without good water he felt he could not achieve this.

In our modern civilized life it becomes increasingly impossible to avoid having chlorine and fluorine in our tap water. When I have met with very heavy chemical treatment of water during my travels, I have gone to the expense of purchasing bottled spring water for my children and animals rather than poison their blood with unnatural chemicals. I buy water in glass bottles. Plastic bottles are known to have adverse effects on health.

Drinking water, put out for dogs, should be changed twice daily. Water dishes or troughs should be placed in shady places. Collect all possible rain-water so long as this has not fallen through factory- or chimney-polluted air, i.e. so long as it is clean rain-water. Beware also of rain-water from near to nuclear plants and pollution from vehicle fumes from heavy traffic.

Do not allow drinking immediately after meals for this washes down the food in a semi-digested state into the lower intestines, causing indigestion and bloating. Puppies require water from an early age. They are thirsty for water long before weaning; they therefore should be provided with shallow dishes of water as soon as their eyes have opened. They will seek and lick up dew from grass and plants; this should be encouraged. This intake of water by pups also helps the nursing bitch to conserve her breast milk.

MISCELLANEOUS CANINE FOODS

HONEY I believe I could not successfully rear domestic dogs without this remarkable antiseptic food. It is of course not a normal item of diet for the carnivores, but the lion enjoys honey and it is considered a staple food of the vegetarian bear, one of the strongest of the wild animals. Honey is the greatest of the natural energizers, a nerve tonic and a supreme heart tonic; indeed it is the only known heart stimulant which is not a drug. Predigested by its makers, the bees, it is absorbed immediately into the bloodstream of the consumer. A diet of milk and honey only can sustain life for months in humans and animals. It has been well and longtime proved that honey is also highly medicinal and will inhibit growth of harmful bacteria in the entire digestive tract and destroy those of a toxic nature.

Hippocrates, called 'the father of all medicine', the great Greek herbalist doctor of ancient times, had two basic remedies with which he cured the sick of almost all their ills. His first remedy was hydromel – honey and water; his second was oxymel – honey and vinegar.

In the famous Frauenfelden Home in Switzerland, sickly infants are placed on a prolonged diet of milk and honey, usually for many weeks, with remarkably good results. The mother of Hillary, the New Zealand beekeeper whose extraordinary stamina enabled him to achieve the first ascent of Mount Everest, together with Sherpa Tensing, in 1953, declared that her son's exceptional strength is much due to the big amounts of honey on which he was reared. The purity of all honey used cannot be over-emphasized. In Europe synthetic honey is a popular article; it has none of the good properties of bee honey and is also bad for the teeth. Purchase honey preferably direct from beekeepers or from health food stores, and get a guarantee that the honey has not come from areas where fruit trees or plants are sprayed with poisonous insecticides. The honey should not be filtered or heat treated; the latter is often done to commercial honey to facilitate the easy pouring of honey into small jars. Therefore it is often best to buy honey in bulk in large cans or jars to safeguard against heat treatment, which destroys 50 per cent of the natural health properties of honey.

In Galilee, Israel, just as I provided medicinal herbs for my goats, dogs, and my own family, I grew a herb garden of special bee herbs. The bees themselves are natural herbalists, and will gorge themselves on bitter rue or pungent lavender and rosemary in preference to garden roses and other merely ornamental flowers (whereas they seek out the wild roses very keenly). The honey provided from the herb garden was naturally very healthful, and buyers came for it from most distant places, and the bees themselves enjoyed excellent health and possessed complete resistance to the many diseases afflicting the local white-sugar-fed bees.

Feed honey to puppies with their milk meal, and to sick dogs either in their water, if they will take it, or in balls of thick honey pushed down their throats. Honey can also be used externally for treatment of burns (see Scalds, p.246).

EGGS Eggs from hens, ducks, or turtles are a rich source of mineral salts and vitamins. The shells given in small amounts, pounded into powder by means of a flat stone, are a good form of giving natural calcium to the dog and are a fine aid to the building of well-textured bone. Eggshell is rather insoluble, but the strong digestive juices of the *healthy* dog can cope with it. Breeders, on my recommendation, have been using successfully this natural bone-building aid for many years now. It is important to make your own eggshell powder. Do not buy stale commercialized eggshell sold expensively as 'Nature-food' or something similar: find out what it contains. Such commercial eggshell, being stale, can endanger by adhering to the inner lining of the digestive tract. Use eggshell as little as you would use salt. Eggs must be fresh, as staleness renders them indigestible. They should be fed raw, because cooking causes them to adhere to the digestive tract. Feed one egg on alternate days per week to adult dogs and likewise to puppies. Eggs are quite a natural food to the dog, for dogs will seek out and eat the eggs of sea-birds and other birds, such as game-birds, which lay their eggs on the ground. Eggs are a very *unsuitable* food for sick animals because of their highly fermentative properties. During the heat of fever, for instance, they rapidly poison the body instead of strengthening it. Egg-and-milk has long been the most misguided of the orthodox medical-recommended invalid foods; the giving of such food has done about as much to spoil cures by orthodox treatment as has the popular use of the destructive sulphonamide group of drugs. It is claimed that raw egg-white harms health: I do not agree. Egg-stealers such as foxes, weasels, cats and rats keep very well, thank you!

SEAWEED Seaweed could be classified with the herbs, but its special properties are so important to canine health that it merits a separate mention. Seaweed is without equal as a source of natural iodine, concerning which substance Lillian R. Carque, ScD, writing in an American journal, states:

Iodine is highly desirable for pregnant mothers. It is especially needed at the age of adolescence for the development of the reproductive organs, particularly in the female in whom the change-over takes place more rapidly than in the male. Adequate iodine also ensures luxuriant hair and skin health; lack gives rise to a very dry skin and loss of hair. Increased iodine intake permits better digestion and assimilation of fatty elements in foods. Organic iodine – the only kind the thyroid gland can appropriate – causes better retention and utilization of calcium and phosphorus; lesser degrees of thyroid deficiency produce bone changes analogous to that of rickets weaknesses. Organic iodine is very essential, too, in combating disease germs and their poisonous excretions. The secretions of the thyroid gland are definitely germicidal. Organic iodine raises the red blood-cell count and has a direct influence on the formation of red blood corpuscles. Ages ago Greek gladiators used seaweed as part of their diet. Certain tribes of American Indians were known to make annual trips to the coast to obtain seaweed, doubtless because they appreciated the therapeutic value in arresting disease. Present-day peasants of the Greek islands make much use of salads of raw seaweed dressed with oil and vinegar. Seaweed, a natural sea food, contains no drug principle or stimulant, and is of far greater value in mineral and vitamin content than is much earth-grown produce raised on impoverished soil.

Seaweed is not an unnatural food for dogs. They would

get this from the intestinal contents of herbivorous animals who will eat it in small amounts. As seaweed gives dark pigment to eyes, nose, and claws, its use is much acclaimed in the canine world. But no doubt its true fame is due to its powers to stimulate hair growth; and through being a glandular tonic, it also stimulates general forward and stalwart body development and promotes strong bones. I am pleased to have been responsible for introducing and popularizing this wonderful product of Nature among dog breeders throughout the world. I have pioneered this also for cattle, goats, sheep, and poultry. Also for all racing livestock, from horses and greyhounds to pigeons. I first introduced seaweed to the veterinary world when a student in the early 1930s; *it was scorned then, but now it is in very popular use worldwide*. Only make sure that the seaweed you use is from safe sources, not polluted sea-shore rubbish.

CAROB   I am very interested in popularizing carob pods as a beneficial food and health aid for dogs, just as I pioneered, long ago, the use of seaweed for dogs. Carob is the fruit of the carob tree, also called locust tree and St John's tree (the pods being called St John's bread because John the Baptist was supposed to have lived on them as a mono-diet for years, as did many of the ancient Jewish rabbis when in hiding from Roman soldiers). A fruit which can sustain life for years is obviously an important one, and so far this one has not been sprayed with pesticide chemicals.

Carob is rich in natural sugars and has all the principal minerals and viatmins. Dogs like to eat it. If pups are fed the pods when young they will continue to eat them when adult dogs. My Afghans eat carob regularly, skilfully spitting out the pips. Remove the sharp point from the top of the pod before giving to the dog.

I have added powdered carob to my puppy and junior meal

formula as a protection against hip dysplasia, and very successful results are obtained.

That ages-old Nature Food, carob, has in recent years been subjected to 'intensive' tests on laboratory animals and our modern scientists have condemned carob as harmful and added its good name to their long list of condemned herbal things. Ignore their ridiculous lists: rely on the experience of the ages.

COCONUT This is another important nature food I am pioneering for dogs and cats and fortunately they thoroughly enjoy it. White of egg and coconut are two foods which supply the important substance albumen (very good for the blood corpuscles).

Coconut is rich in digestible oils and also provides fibre which passes out of the body and takes with it any worms' eggs. It should be fed on its own, added to cereals, not mixed into commercial foods as it turns rancid quite quickly and could spoil other foods. Fortunately, like carob, coconuts are rarely sprayed with chemicals as their hard shells resist insect damage.

One dessertspoon of desiccated coconut, three or four days a week, is the amount for an average size dog, but less should be given to cats.

AVOCADO PEAR Raw, peeled and mashed, this gives a vital oil.

OLIVES Black (but not green) olives, with stones removed, are excellent mashed up with cereals. Their oil is recommended. Make sure olive produce is not from chemically-sprayed trees. Modern olive groves are frequently sprayed with insecticide chemicals. Remember that green olives are unripe black olives.

FINAL NOTES

Dogs should never have their natural instincts thwarted in the matter of diet. They should not be prevented from eating the droppings from grass-fed cattle and horses, from which they can get many vital elements derived from the herbage on which the animals have grazed and in a form easily assimilated by the dog. Likewise, puppies should not be prevented from eating earth, sand and small stones. These remove intestinal impurities and worms in the same way as couch-grass eating, which should also be encouraged. Only eating of its own or other dogs' faeces is a depraved habit and should be checked at once.

To complete this chapter, I am giving in detail the Natural Rearing Puppy and Adult Dog Diets which, when in *proper* daily use, have banished all disease from dogs. This has been well proved during the past fifty years by kennels in all parts of the world. Adequate exercise and hygienic kennelling are also of importance to achieve this total health. When dog owners have obtained this health among their own dogs, it is hoped they will extend their knowledge to the other animals, cats, cattle, horses, poultry, and so forth and, of greater importance, to the rearing of their childen, who also require a basic diet of uncooked natural foods and freedom from the use of chemical medicines and vaccines.

But before giving the diets, I want to mention a question which so often reaches me: Can dogs be reared on a vegetarian diet? Yes, they can be so reared. But as I am writing this book on Natural Rearing, I do not want to deal with the unnatural here. A vegetarian diet of whole (mostly raw) foods, given in addition to whole-grain cereals, eggs, cheese, milk and pulses for protein, can keep a dog in good health, but such diet is far more difficult to feed successfully than the natural carnivorous one. However, there are many vegetarian dog owners who are loth to feed meat, and for this reason I have written a booklet, *Healthy Vegetarian Dogs and Cats*, obtainable from Natural Rearing Products' agencies.

The Natural Rearing Diets given below have been in use for a *very* long time and it is they which mostly have made those two words 'Natural Rearing' popular words among dog owners of many lands. They have created a big demand for NR stock and NR has come to signify truly sound health.

NATURAL REARING PUPPY DIET

Puppies reared according to the laws of Nature are always far superior in every way to stock incorrectly reared on the usual unnatural canine diets, and have been found to possess an extraordinary resistance to all disease. Natural Rearing gives exceptionally strong bone, dense body hair, heavy muscle in place of fat, and always sound nerves. The usual puppy ailments do not occur when Natural Rearing is strictly followed. Puppies may pick up from unclean ground the eggs of round worms excreted by other puppies, and these will develop, but they will be expelled in time and there will be no infestation. The four main rules of Natural Rearing are: (1) correct natural diet of raw foods; (2) abundant sunlight and fresh air; (3) at least two hours' exercise daily (including plenty of running exercise) and this to be outside kennel enclosures; (4) hygenic kennelling, with the use of earth and grass runs to give contact with the vital radiations of the earth. No concrete runs should be used. But the old-fashioned brick or cobblestones, with good drainage provided, can be utilized on very damp land; gravel, likewise, can be used very well as it can be dug up and replaced with new when it has become unclean from over-use. Couch grass (dog-grass, twitch) should be planted outside, near kennel runs, for medicinal use of dogs.

Natural Rearing Diet (from weaning to four months)

For average breed puppy. For big breeds and toy breeds, increase or decrease accordingly. No puppy should be given other than the dam's milk food before four weeks of age. Other milky foods can then be given if desired. It is impossible to give exact quantities. All puppies of all breeds differ in appetite capacity. Never give hot food or refrigerated very cold food – blood heat (tepid) or normal cold is natural. Hot food damages the stomach and intestines and can cause cancer. Animals usually, wisely, refuse to touch hot or very cold food. Provide plenty of fresh drinking water day and night. Avoid plastic dishes.

8 a.m.: Fluid meal of raw milk (cow or goat), not dried or canned or long-life milk, strengthened with honey and tree-barks' blend gruel. (A blend of nutritious barks of trees, roots and cereals; my own Natural Rearing formula. See p. 320.) *Less than half pint*.

12 noon: Whole-grain flaked porridge oats, wheat, barley, or rye, or mixed flakes, soaked overnight in cold milk (sour milk is excellent for this), and a few finely chopped raisins, a teaspoonful of desiccated coconut. Alternatively, the cereal flakes can be soaked in cabbage or nettle water. Barley, being the most digestible of the cereals, should be used for weaning if available. A perfect cereal meal for growing puppies is two parts barley flakes to one part oat flakes (such as sold in packets for porridge making), soaked in fresh cold milk. *Use one large handful of flaked cereal or cereals*. With this meal two or three slices of stale wholewheat bread should be given. When biscuits or meal are preferred, use only chemical-free,

44

farmhouse type of 'health' biscuit, a blend of true whole-grain cereals. If it is desired to feed fruit to the puppy – finely grated apple is a healthful food – it should be mixed in with flaked cereals and milk. There is now available a blend of four cereals and herbs made to my formula (in a Norfolk windmill). Add a small teaspoon of oil. This is especially needed in long-coat breeds, but all breeds need some oil. I consider the only *safe* oils nowadays to be sesame, corn (maize) or sunflower.

4 p.m.: Meat: approximately two ounces raw, shredded (cow or horse flesh, or breast of mutton – the soft mutton bones may be given). Meat should never be minced, pups' powerful stomach muscles should be used for meat digestion; after ten weeks of age, meat should be given in pieces about the size of a £1 coin, increasing in size to pieces as large as a walnut after four months. Raw, finely cut herrings sprinkled with flaked oats can be fed once or twice weekly as a change from meat. Scald the fish well to soften it before cutting. Rabbit meat may also be given; dogs thoroughly enjoy it. Unless caught fresh it should be softened in hot water.

8 p.m.: (main meal) Meat: approximately two ounces (as above).

Bones must be given with meat – meat without bones is unnatural.

Plus one teaspoonful wheat germ (such as Bemax, Froment, etc), and equal amount of bran for extra roughage. When bran is not available, a sprinkle of flaked cereals can be used.

Plus one teaspoonful cod-liver oil (in winter), olive oil (in summer).

Plus a sprinkle of seaweed powder (rich in natural minerals, especially iodine) (see p. 320), promotes dense body hair, strengthens nerves.

Plus one teaspoonful raw green leaves: dandelion, clover, parsley, mint, watercress, nasturtium, celery, or mallow (young) leaves; a mixture of several is good. The leaves must be finely chopped with a sharp knife, almost to a pulp, as dogs have difficulty in digesting cellulose.

The daily ration of green food is essential to health   Raw chopped onion, one teaspoonful, is also excellent, especially when worms or skin disorders are present. Two or three herbal antiseptic tablets, of such herbs as garlic, rue, eucalyptus, etc are recommended several days weekly. Raw eggs on meat occasionally, or raw eggs can be given on the cereal food. It may be necessary to make an incision with a knife on the meat, to prevent the dog from shaking off the supplements, which should be rubbed in. Or use a sprinkle of cold water to make the supplements adhere.

Most adult dogs love dried fruits, especially figs and raisins. Both are much used in the Middle East for salukis and others.

After four months, omit the 8 a.m. feeding, and feed only at 12 noon, 4 p.m., and 8 p.m. The cereal allowance should be increased, fully to satisfy appetite, the meat to eight ounces or more, and the raw vegetable to one dessertspoon. After eight months, meals should be reduced to two: cereal at midday; meat in the evening, sufficient food being given each meal to satisfy.

Note   Every puppy, from weaning onward, should rest and cleanse its internal organs frequently by fasts on plain water only. A puppy should never be coaxed or tempted to eat. If food is not eaten rapidly the puppy should be fasted for twelve hours or more. Every puppy over four months old should have a half-day fast one day per week (suggested every Sunday); a whole-day fast one day per month; every adult a weekly one-day fast.

Do not prevent puppies from eating earth or excreta from grass-fed cattle, etc, as this is natural to carnivores. Also encourage them to eat grass.

Important Throughout this scientific diet, meat and starch foods should not be mixed up in quantity at the same meal. They are incompatible and cause scouring, with resultant indigestion, which is the root of hysteria, gastritis, worms, and other disorders. The only exception is the sprinkle of flaked oats (a protein-rich cereal) to supply extra roughage if bran is not available, or a hard-baked wholewheat crust or biscuit as a finish, to promote saliva flow. Also plain milk should not be given in large amounts; it should be fortified with honey or thickened with tree bark flour or whole-grain cereals, thus overcoming the tendency to create mucus. Precautions should be taken against the feeding of soured foods (cereals) during hot weather. Sour food can cause serious intestinal illness. Cooked meat also sours, whereas raw meat only ripens.

The diet given herewith is for show stock and can be simplified for everyday use.

Further note The quantities given are for average puppies; larger breed puppies require far greater quantities of food, according to size.

So many people write to me for details of correct amounts to give puppies. I have always declined to supply such information, for so much is dependent upon so many variable factors: breed, build of puppy, quality of food, amount of exercise being given, even the temperament of the puppy in question. Also, it must be understood that growing stock needs more daily food than adult. However, for those persons insistent on feeding by weighed-out amounts, I think that Stonehenge's observations are the soundest that I have yet met with in any canine book.

The quantity by weight which is received by the growing puppy is from one-twelfth to one-twentieth of the weight of its body, varying with the rapidity of growth and a good deal with the breed also. Thus a twelve-pound dog will take from five-eighths of a pound to a pound of food, and a twenty-six-pound dog from two to three pounds. When they arrive at full growth, more than the smaller of these weights is very seldom wanted, and it may be taken as the average lot of food of this kind for all dogs in tolerably active exercise.

Stonehenge advocates a raw flesh and cooked cereal diet for dog rearing. However, I think that a dog should be allowed to eat to capacity on plain whole-grain cereals, only controlling the amount of meat. A dog could well overeat on meat, but is unlikely to do so on plain cereals.

Another simple method of calculation is based on the ancient Arab teaching that the human body requires no more than two to three pounds of food per day for health. This basic amount can be reduced according to the size of the dog in question, though remember that the dog takes more active exercise, thus using up more food; it was on this teaching that I based the food needs of my Afghan hounds.

One final comment applicable to all puppies is: give puppies as much of natural foods as they will eat up keenly without their stomachs becoming distended after eating.

A word of advice about adult dogs: do not be too emphatic or dogmatic about such things as hours of feeding and sticking exactly to the diet. The habits and likes of the individual dog or cat should be respected. My own Afghans and many other Afghans and salukis, in their age-old wisdom, do not like to eat when the weather turns hot; in summer even meat will be refused so I delay the midday cereal/milk meal until late afternoon, often as late as 5 p.m. As I keep this meal well separated from the meat meal – except for allowing a whole-wheat biscuit or rusk and a few dried figs or dates before meat so as to line the stomach against sharp bones – it is often very late at night before the meat is fed. Inconvenient for me, but healthful for the dogs; and summer heat does not last the year through! After all, carnivores are night hunters and eaters by nature, so I am merely following what is natural.

Animals, of course, have food likes and dislikes. My Afghans, for instance, generally prefer their cereal flakes almost dry. They do not like the milk poured over the flakes so I provide two plates at this meal. One consists of flaked cereals with extra herbal bran made more palatable by the addition of dried coconut (one dessertspoon per hound), a half dessertspoon of *tahina* (prepared, crushed sesame seeds) and some raisins, the raisins on the side so that they can be chewed better. The second plate is of milk lightly thickened with a sprinkle of bran and some cereal flakes and/or meal, but it is essentially a liquid dish.

For the night meat meal, see the diet. If I feed sprouted grains and pulses, they are minced fine and given with the meat as an extra to the finely-cut salad greens. Eggs are also better on the meat because they help the extras to adhere to it.

SPECIMEN DIET FOR AN AVERAGE SIZE ADULT DOG

Midday: 100 per cent flaked whole-grain wheat, rye, or barley, softened with either raw milk or vegetable juice. I have made available a four-cereals flake meal with herbs, popular with all dogs. Sour milk is excellent with this. Wholewheat, rye, or corn bread, or biscuits of same, also (uncooked) wholemaize flour, can be added to this meal. Raw eggs can

49

also be mixed into the cereal, approximately four times per week. Likewise, some corn (maize) or sunflower oil, or sesame (*tahina*), one teaspoon for an average size dog; use far less if the dog is fat.

Note No adult dog should be fed before midday; the hours from midnight to midday are strongly eliminative ones. In-between-meal scraps are harmful. However, hunting breeds of greyhound build, with small stomachs, often want an early-morning meal instead of at midday.

Evening (main feed): Meat, raw, in large pieces, never minced. Very hard-frozen meat is as harmful as cooked meat. A small quantity of fat should be included. Give raw bones.
  Plus one teaspoon wheat-germ flakes.
  Plus one teaspoon cod-liver oil (winter).
  Plus seaweed powder.
  Plus one heaped dessertspoon very finely chopped raw green herb, such as parsley, watercress, dandelion, celery (young), mustard (young), chickweed, goosegrass (cleavers), purslane, cresses (all kinds). The inclusion of the herb is important. Grated raw carrot can also be added.
  Plus several dessertspoons of bran or flaked oats to replace lost roughage of the skin and hair.
  When bones are given, they should be raw only, and fed after the meat. They should not be given on an empty stomach.

In-whelp bitches, nursing bitches, and invalid adults are permitted an early-morning meal of milk and honey; a dessertspoon of bran can be added to prevent mucus formation; also tree-barks' flour to be added. When available, grapes or apples, pressed through cheese-cloth or through strong muslin, make a good addition to this morning drink.
  All the carnivorous animals need at least one meatless day

per week and one day on fluids only, i.e. four or five days only of meat feeding. No wild dog would be able to kill prey every day of every week. Appreciating this fact, most of the zoos of the world fast the carnivores – lions, tigers, wolves – one day each week.

For the Natural Rearing diet it is recommended there be one meatless day per week, using instead milk, eggs, white cheese with whole-grain cereals, rice, cooked pulses such as beans, lentils, etc. One fast day should follow this, giving fluids only and a laxative the same night, also herbal pills the next morning. This simple Nature treatment wards off disease toxins, rests the kidneys, which are always over-worked on a meat diet, and rejuvenates the dog. Hungry dogs can be given a little honey in their water at meal times, or very watery diluted milk, or water from flaked oats or barley, obtained from pouring medium-hot water over the flakes and soaking them overnight.

Note An increasing demand in England, America and Canada for natural, whole-grain cereals has made such products as wheat, barley, rye, corn, etc, available in most towns, at many co-operative stores, health food stores, etc. Many mills supply direct by mail. The address of the current suppliers of Natural Rearing products of all kinds is on page 320.

In the USA and Canada, natural, flaked cereals of many kinds are now obtainable from the widespread health food stores. But make sure they are not 'toasted' after flaking. This is often done to ensure long life, but the high-heat treatment kills much of the health properties of the cereals.

HERBAL PILLS *Make sure* your supply is a reliable and safe one. There is no guarantee, except personal knowledge of the management of the firm whose pills you are buying, that good quality *fresh* herbs are being used in their products. There is no control to prevent firms from buying up stale 'remainder' herbs and using them in their products. The modern popularity of herbs has attracted the unscrupulous: take care.

PILLS DOSAGE Do not over-dose. When dogs are on a course of herbal pills, do not give a daily dose seven days of every week. Dose for five days only of the seven, otherwise the body becomes too accustomed to the pills and they lose their healing power as a result. Also give different, alternative herbal remedies from time to time.

2

Care of the Brood Bitch

My half century of veterinary medicine work has revealed to me the appalling amount of canine disease prevalent today in all parts of the world. Nearly 50 per cent of such disease is hereditary and will require drastic and long-term measures wholly to breed-out from the various strains in which it is manifest. But the other 50 per cent is readily preventable and curable by promptly and wholeheartedly adopting Natural Rearing (NR) rules. The dog is a most simple animal to keep in good health. It has not the complicated digestive system of the human being, for instance, which makes health maintenance or disease cure such a far more involved and long-term business; any child can keep a dog in great health; and yet – because unnatural rearing methods are the rule – the amount of canine disease prevalent in the civilized world today is a horrible thought. To comprehend present-day canine disease, one has only to read through modern veterinary medical textbooks and to study the long lists of ailments which afflict a species of animal, whose anatomy and way of life should by rights enable it to be the healthiest of all domestic animals. Such unpleasant reading must give one reason for thought.

I have written the puppy-rearing section to ensure that all puppies should be given the chance of enjoying their rightful inheritance of good health. When all puppies are reared by such methods, canine disease will positively disappear within a very few generations of NR stock. Such has been my own experience, and the experience of leading breeders in England and overseas. The words of Mrs Wingfield Digby – pioneer Keeshond breeder and owner of the famous Van Zaadam Keeshonds in England – are apt. Writing of NR stock, she says: 'Never before have I seen such forward and intelligent puppies. It is as if they felt extra well.'

The international hounds expert and author of canine books, Herr P.M.C. Toepel of Holland, wrote about the first NR Afghans he ever saw, two black Afghan male pups at a championship show in England. They so attracted his attention that he made enquiries and was told they were raised by a 'new' method (it must have been in the early 1930s). Herr Toepel was greatly impressed by the unusual vitality of the Afghan pups and gave them both high awards. They were from the first NR litter I ever raised.

The care of the in-whelp bitch is almost totally neglected in most dog-breeding establishments. The bitch is merely mated and then expected to produce her litter at the end of the nine-weeks' period; no changes in diet or general treatment have been followed at all. In the rare cases when the in-whelp bitch is singled out for special attention, the treatment is generally of a most unnatural nature. There is usually over-feeding, resulting in heavy, inactive puppies, which cause whelping difficulties. Dosage with chemical calcium is supposed to 'grow' strong bone, but in fact acts as a kidney irritant and causes unnatural brittleness of the bony structure of the body (also causes rigidity of the bone parts of the litter in embryo, thus making further whelping difficulties).

Such neglect of the in-whelp bitch is remarkable when it must be appreciated that the health of the forthcoming litter is much affected by the dam throughout the nine-weeks' in-whelp period. In actual fact, the health of a litter of puppies is 50 per cent dependent on prenatal care and diet.

The Arabs say, concerning their famous Arabian horses, that the stallion gives type to the foals, the mare gives *health*. They pay endless attention to the health of their brood mares. The same care is necessary for the brood bitch from puppy-hood, if she is to produce when adult a litter truly healthy and capable of improving the health standard of the breed.

Dr G.T. Wrench, in his important book concerning that natural-living race of people, the Hunza tribe of the Indian mountains, goes even further than my statement concerning the effect of prenatal health on the offspring. He states: 'Unless the mother is healthy and carries healthy blood to her conception, the wholeness of health cannot be attained.' And yet how many bitches are mated year after year when in a state of actual disease: sufferers of skin diseases, kidney diseases, obesity, glandular ailments, and many other sub-health conditions? No wonder that such bitches prove barren, or whelp litters which fade away at birth or are carried off by one or another of the so-called epidemic diseases shortly after weaning, especially the modern parvovirus. Or if litters bred from unhealthy stock do survive, such stock is malformed with 'shelly' bone, bent, rickety limbs and sparse hair, or very subject to worm infestation, or are constant sufferers from one or more of the canine ailments which have long been looked upon as being the normal lot of the canine race.

Appreciating that good bone formation, nerve structure, and hair growth are dependent upon the blood of the dam during the all-important nine weeks of growth in the womb, it is understandable that in any book concerned with puppy rearing, a chapter on care of the in-whelp bitch is essential.

As for the stud dog, good health should again be an essential when making a choice of sire, for through the stud dog, just as with the brood bitch, hereditary ailments can enter and dominate the future lives of the unborn puppies.

The mange-type of skin disease prevalent in many strains of chows and dachshunds; chorea in collies and terriers; kidney disease in Scottish terriers; hind-quarters paralysis in dachshunds and Pekinese; hip disease (hip dysplasia) in Alsatians, Labradors, and Samoyeds; slipped stifle joint in King Charles spaniels and poodles; epileptic fits in Kerry blues; deafness in bull terriers, juvenile blindness in Afghans, and middle-aged blindness in Border collies – these are but a few examples to be found of hereditary diseases in the hitherto healthy canine race; and perhaps the miniature and toy poodles are the worst of all examples of man's unnatural rearing methods, suffering as they do from such inherited ailments as toothlessness, deformed inner ears, and blindness. Then there are among many breeds general epilepsy, chronic skin diseases, heart diseases, diabetes, and so on, and latterly there is widespread cancer, all greatly established by vaccinations from stock made artificially diseased in laboratories. Such ailments can now be bred out only with infinite patience and trouble.

As Miss Peggy E. Brown, of Harrogate, who studied agriculture at Reading University, writes:

Without a doubt it is this everlasting breeding for show points at the expense of all else that is the cause of all the degeneration in canine health. If the things that matter, principally good health, are never bred for, they are *bound* to get lost. It only needs one champion dog to be popular at stud and yet suffering with some serious hereditary ailment, and in no time it will spread right through a breed. Just look how wonderful are the Border collies – bred for stamina, intelligence, etc, yet never for looks to a Show Standard, nor are they inoculated; yet, despite no Show Standard, they are easily recognizable as a breed, in type. *They* are not wiped out by modern diseases, and they get the roughest, but reasonably nourishing, food, from poultry and pig meal to milk. With some raw meat also, they would become superb. Nothing beyond their reach.

These collies do get a limited amount of meat at certain seasons, dead lambs, carcasses of dead sheep, also entrails of rabbits. Some farmers have a superstitious belief against feeding meat to collies in case they turn 'killers'. But I have been much with Border collies and have seen them dig up and eat, or salvage from rivers, sheep carcasses. However, I note sadly that Peggy Brown's praise of the healthy Border collie (and I too know the breed well on the moorlands of the Pennine Hills, in northern England) was written for the second edition of my *Canine Herbal*, in 1963, and as I revise this sixth edition in late 1990, the health of this stalwart breed has declined like most of the other breeds, influenced in this case by farm foods having lost their wholesome naturalness and become largely shop-bought and devitalized. In a recent BBC 'News from Wales' programme, it was stated that the working collie does not get just treatment and that, although its daily work saves the farmer hundreds of pounds in labour weekly, the collie is unlikely to have £5 spared towards the purchase of good food weekly in reward for such important work. There is now widespread inherited eye disease in Border collies, ending in total blindness, unbearably tragic in a working breed whose efficiency much depends on keen sight.

It is a logical consideration, therefore, that the health of a stud dog should be carefully considered when making a selection for breeding; it is of equal importance (of greater importance in my opinion) with show points. Anyway, show merit is largely dependent on good bone formation, hair growth, true movement, all of which are, in turn, largely dependent on sound health. In most breeds (the dog being a carnivorous animal) good strong jaw formation is a desirable show point; growth of jaw is largely determined by good rearing.

In addition to ensuring that a bitch is in the highest possible state of health at the time of mating, the period of the year at which the litter will be born should also be taken into consideration. Spring litters are natural, winter litters unnatural. It is noticeable that newly imported breeds, which have come from lands where they have been allowed to lead a natural, often semi-wild, life, seldom come on heat more than once a year. The females of that hardy wild animal, the jackal, closely related to the dog family (indeed they will mate with dogs), come into season only once a year. They mate for life and remain entirely loyal to one mate. In dog breeding, bitches should be allowed to mate with dogs for which they show preference. They should never be forced to mate with a disliked dog merely because that dog has good blood lines.

Horse breeders wisely place a far higher value on spring-born foals. It is the opinion of the horse world that winter-born foals never attain the stamina of the spring-born.

The milk-feeding question here plays a part. In the spring when cattle are grazing on the new grass, the milk is far better in every way than winter milk. Indeed, winter milk from cows or goats is not a suitable puppy-weaning food at all.

Menstruation, or 'on heat', is also a partial cleansing of the body. The reproductive organs are areas of the body which frequently become very toxin laden in wrongly reared animals. The on-heat period of a healthy bitch is short and there is no evil-smelling discharge whatsoever. In such cases it is purely an outflow of the organs of reproduction in preparation for mating and subsequent birth; there is only a short cleansing process. Feed the bitch on a lighter diet than usual when on heat. Give less meat. Give the special female herbs which will also be used if she is mated and thus made in-whelp. The best-known female herbs are wild raspberry leaves, chamomile, feverfew, elder flower, rose hips, artemesia (southernwood).

DIET FOR THE IN-WHELP BITCH

The rule of paramount importance in diet for the in-whelp bitch is, of course, feed *raw* foods. The previous chapter described how cooking causes general deterioration of the entire digestive system, from the teeth to the lowermost region of the bowels. Cooked food clogs around the teeth and causes dental decay; also weakness of jaw formation, owing to the bones and muscles of the jaws being insufficiently exercised because of the feeding of heat-softened pappy foods; canned foods are yet worse. The digestive juices are weakened, because cooked food is semi-digested in the process of cooking, and therefore the powerful digestive juices, natural to the dog, are no longer fully required or utilized. The powerful muscles of stomach and intestines, with which the carnivorous races are so well supplied (the digestive juices and intestinal muscles can break down and partially dissolve such hard substances as lumps of bone, skin and hair, pieces of gristle, and so on), in their turn weaken and diminish. They – as with the digestive juices – being deprived of their rightful work, and being insufficiently utilized – just as with an injured limb kept in splints for a lengthy time – become flabby and eventually shrivel. Therefore, for the unborn litter to be properly nourished, the bitch's diet must be mainly raw foods, only a little semi-cooked cereal food being the exception to the rule. Often around the fourth week the bitch will refuse her food and give herself a voluntary fast. This is very frequent and is due to digestive disturbances caused by her condition. She should never be coaxed to eat at such times. At the most she should be offered a raw milk-honey diet. Normal appetite will soon return, and the bitch is generally found to have developed an increased appetite.

It will soon be found that a healthy bitch requires far less food than an unhealthy one. When I think back on the enormous quantities of food that I used to feed my dogs when I was a schoolgirl and university student, and generally I had two or three dogs in my care, I am always left amazed at the recollection. The diet for my borzoi dog, for instance, used to be almost a bucketful of soaked white houndmeal, with lumps of cooked meat supplied with it. The dog used to eat this vast daily feed, but he never fattened and was always ailing with eczema and kindred diseases – and no wonder! My Afghan hounds have attained great height and condition on a general daily ration of 1¼lb of raw meat four or five days per week, and ½lb of whole-grain cereal. Actually, the Essenes, that great sect of Eastern people, unsurpassed doctors, used to rule that no adult human being should consume more than 2lb of food daily, for true health. This fact makes one wonder, when the huge quantities of food which breeders give daily to their dogs are taken into consideration. The real solution is that healthy bodies utilize every particle of food fed to them, whereas unhealthy bodies in the main allow most of the food fed to them to pass through the intestines only semi-digested, and therefore *twice the normal quantities of food have to be fed to the unhealthy animals* in order to prevent excessive thinness and other subnormal health conditions resulting from underfeeding.

A great mistake is made when double-ration feeding of the in-whelp bitch is practised, the idea behind such feeding being that the unborn and rapidly developing litter must be well and sufficiently nourished. The idea is entirely erroneous, and if practised is truly harmful, causing sour food deposits to accumulate in the intestines, and furthermore putting an additional burden on the bloodstream which is already overworked at such times, dealing with the excretions from the rapidly growing litter of puppies which, while in the womb, utilize the bloodstream of the dam in order to remove their own waste products. An in-whelp bitch requires extra milk for calcium provision; extra intake of water is also required to flush out the kidneys, which also bear part of the burden of ridding the body of the excretions of the developing litter. Clean water must always be available, day and night. Indeed, increased thirst is a good indication that a bitch is pregnant.

Further attention should be paid to an abundant supply of natural mineral salts – supplied in the daily ration of raw green herbs, whole-grain cereals, and, to some extent, by the raw meat. For this purpose I have evolved a formula giving the minerals most rich in vegetation of land and sea, carefully dried and powdered: nettles, comfrey and seaweed, all blended into a powder for giving on the raw meat. This natural mineral powder (NR seaweed blend), fed daily to the bitch throughout the nine-weeks' in-whelp period, gives amazing results, not only in general improvement of the litter, but in overcoming such in-whelp ailments as streptococcal infection, acid or failing milk, and so forth.

Special attention must be paid to the diet immediately before whelping. The litter has ceased growing by the beginning of the eighth week, external furnishing such as nails and hair being mainly the only developments, and in general the puppies are very restless and active in preparation for the leaving of the womb. At such a time the organism of the dam does not want to be burdened with much food digestion; a gentle laxative diet should be aimed at for the last week of the in-whelp period. Meat supply should be reduced, and a main meal of raw milk, flaked oats, or barley fed up to one or two days before the actual birth, when the bitch should be placed entirely on a fluid diet, a diet of milk and honey – average quantity is one heaped teaspoon of honey to a large breakfast-cupful of milk. A toy-breed bitch would require on average a small cupful of milk and a half teaspoon of honey twice a day, a large breed about a half pint or more per meal. Any reliable unadulterated make of that wonderful tree-barks' flour food, slippery elm or red elm tree-flour food is a very helpful aid to bitches at such times, and has been utilized by hundreds of breeders always with great success. Such food is also the ideal diet for the two days following whelping, when, as with immediately preceding whelping, no solid food should be given under any circumstances. This feeding of an entirely fluid diet immediately before and after whelping has done an immeasurable amount of good in reducing loss of life through whelping complications. The theory of such a measure is a sound one, it being that when the forces of the body are freed from the necessity of food digestion, they are at liberty for any other purpose of which the body may have need. For instance, during disease treatment, total fasting is employed in order to release the body powers for the processes of the cleansing of the bloodstream and the speedy removal of all disease toxins, and the subsequent repair of body tissues damaged in the interval of disease. In the case of the in-whelp bitch, all the forces of the body can be concentrated on the birth of the puppies, and the prevention of the development of any fever conditions – which sometimes affect bitches not in total health, with the subsequent attack of puerperal fever and other allied ailments of birth.

The body also has much work to do following the whelping, in the production of a good alkaline toxin-free milk flow and the shrinkage to natural size of the stretched organs of birth. There is also the complete expulsion of the products of after-birth to be dealt with.

Mention should be made here of that wonderful aid to easy whelping, the wild raspberry leaf. I was the first to popularize this herb among dog breeders, as long ago as the 1930s; it had never been used hitherto for animals but is now in habitual use as a whelping aid in kennels in all parts of the world. The popularity of the herb grew solely out of results obtained. When hitherto proved difficult whelpers whelped normal litters easily and speedily, following treatment with the herb, it was understandable that breeders should spread the news far and wide. In my veterinary-treatment files I have hundreds of reports from breeders supplying details of hitherto undreamt-of successful whelpings, especially from owners of the notoriously difficult whelping breeds, such as most of the toy breeds. The action of the herb on the organs of reproduction is mainly tonic; hence its further use for sluggish stud dogs. The North American Indians, gypsies, and other races with a profound knowledge of herbal medicine, have long prescribed raspberry-leaf brew as an important medicine for pregnant women. A gypsy herbal document advises: 'Let all creatures with young, human and animal, take freely of raspberry herb. They will have very easy "times", and will be saved a tremendous amount of suffering.' Harold Ward, in his book, *Herbal Manual* (for humans), states: 'Thompson and his immediate successors strongly advised the free drinking of raspberry-leaves' infusion for several months before confinement as an aid to parturition, and it is still in much demand.'

My book has no space for publication in detail of breeders' reports – the book would grow to impossible length – but the use of raspberry leaf being of such importance to canine well-being and the birthright of every brood bitch, I have made an exception here. Miss Florence Cockayne is an Irish terrier breeder, at Gorton, Suffolk (England), and is a hospital-trained nurse (St Thomas's).

As for raspberry leaves, I've never seen such easy whelpings until I used this herb, and the mothers keep so well during pregnancy, bowel evacuation being perfect. Bitches with their first litters give no trouble, the puppies being whelped effortlessly and with no pain. I sent some raspberry leaves on to a bulldog breeder in New South Wales, and she was absolutely amazed at the results; she had always had such ghastly times with her bitches, some of them sometimes being three days in labour. I had a Pekinese bitch who had had two miscarriages, but after having raspberry brew, carried her puppies full time and hardly knew she was whelping.

Mrs S. Bancroft-Wilson, *Dog World*, England, pug correspondent and breeder of the Longlands pugs, also sent me a typical report: 'I have had wonderful results from the raspberry-leaf herb; breeding as I do from small well-boned bitches, I find the herb causes them to whelp quickly and easily. *I consider it is little short of miraculous*.'

Interest in raspberry herb has had a world revival in recent years; so much so that the very conservative human medical journals have devoted articles to the use of this herb in childbirth, though such articles in the main – as is usually the case when reference to crude herbs is made in the chemical drug-dominated medical journals – were scornful, attesting any alleged merits to the mere psychological sphere of influence.

We who have studied the ways of wild animals know that in springtime they seek out various pregnancy plants, especially the early leaves and shoots of the wild raspberry and wild rose, chamomile, feverfew, and pennyroyal. Springtime is the natural breeding time for animals. The female carnivores, preying on the herb-eating animals and, above all, seeking the herb-rich intestines of their prey, would quite surely get a sufficiency of pregnancy herbs to keep their own reproductive systems in good clean health and aid the birth process of their offspring.

Before leaving the subject of raspberry-leaf herb, it should be mentioned how greatly the herb is associated with the reproductive organs, it being noticed at the time of whelping of bitches treated with raspberry that placentas are often very dark green and, further, that the strong and unmistakable odour of raspberry leaf is present throughout the time of the actual whelping and associated with the birth discharge. Many breeders have commented on this.

However, even raspberry leaf will not produce normal and easy whelping if exercise is neglected. At least two hours' free (unleashed) exercise on clean land is essential throughout the in-whelp months, and frequent daily walks.

Finally, for the best results, the 'three nines' should be known, followed and remembered, for on them is based canine health for the entire lifetime.

The three nines are:

First, the nine weeks from the day of mating until the first week following the birth of the litter. Those nine weeks should be weeks of unceasing natural care.

Second, the nine weeks' care of the litter, their weaning and essential early training.

Third, nine months, not weeks, of the rearing of the pups, their daily diet of natural foods and their daily exercise. In those vital months the future lifetime of good or bad health is created. Ample diet of whole foods means development of ample stomach and intestinal capacity fully to digest foods, a strong bony frame which can never succumb to bone deformities such as hip dysplasia, etc, and strong development of the sexual organs.

If those vital nine months of first growing are made a time of uncaring neglect, no future care, no matter how good and efficient, can ever give total health in adult life.

RETENTION OF PUPPIES

It is general for the carnivores to give birth to their whelps easily and speedily. But sometimes an ill-placed puppy – or in an unhealthy bitch, the whole litter – may be retained. Again, it is of great importance that the in-whelp bitch should be at the peak of good health, for in the case of abnormalities such as this there is then little risk of septic conditions developing. It is usually sufficient to give strong doses of raspberry-leaf herbs at four-hourly intervals for several days: two tablespoons of powdered or finely minced raspberry herb, plus one dessertspoonful of molasses or black treacle, liquefied with sufficient warm water and given to the bitch (by force drenching if necessary, for raspberry is a bitter-tasting herb when given in large doses). In cases of retained puppies, the bitch must be fasted until all are expelled. Semi-fasting is permissible, on a three-meal-per-day diet of milk and honey. In very severe cases of retained whelps, two tablespoons of a brew of pennyroyal herb, plus one tablespoonful of Epsom salts dissolved in the herb brew, should be given as a drench of one small cupful thrice daily. Drinks of linseed tea, given with the milk-honey meals, are helpful.

Since the fourth edition I have used a new formula based on my work with goats in Mexico, where many died every spring birthing their kids. The herbal brew I gave them saved all; there were no more deaths of mothers or kids. The formula is: six ivy leaves, one teaspoon sage, one heaped teaspoon southernwood, one sprig rosemary, four cloves, one pint cold water. Place in pan, cover tightly, heat slowly. Remove before boiling, steep for three hours, do not strain. Give four tablespoons, slowly, every three hours. If no results and the bitch shows much distress and is unable to pass the retained puppies, surgery may be needed.

RETENTION OF AFTERBIRTH

Retention of afterbirth is more common to the cow, goat or ewe than to the dog, as bitches have to pass only small placentas, which leave their bodies easily. But in the case of retention in old bitches or in some species of the toy breeds, a brew made from one to three ivy leaves boiled up in a cupful of cold water, then allowed to brew for two hours, is a proved remedy. I always feed a handful of fresh ivy leaves to every goat as soon as she has given birth to her kid or kids. Dosage of ivy brew is two dessertspoons every three hours. If a bitch shows any discomfort following the birth of puppies, put her on a liquid diet of honey and water, or honey-milk-water, for several days and give laxatives.

DIET OF THE NURSING BITCH

This diet is identical with the in-whelp diet, except for increased rations, now that the bitch is free of the extra excretory burden hitherto imposed upon her by the litter developing within her womb. An additional early-morning meal of fluid food, milk with honey and tree-barks' flour, can be given if the litter is a large one. Oats should form the bulk of the cereal food as they are more breast-milk forming, and have more assimilable and concentrated protein than any other cereal for this purpose.

A healthy bitch should be able to feed her litter – large or small – for nine weeks. The Arabs reckon that a healthy lactation corresponds – at its minimum – to the duration of pregnancy. Thus the bitch will feed her litter for nine weeks or more, the human mother for at least nine months. But on modern unnatural diet a bitch's milk is often failing or acid at four weeks, and the human mother has to resort to devitalizing dried milk for her offspring after only a few months.

TO INCREASE MILK RAPIDLY All of the following foods are known to make milk: unpasteurized cow or goat milk, grated raw carrot, cooked carrot (mashed), oat flakes, wholewheat, rye, beanmeal, seaweed powder (has been proved to increase butterfat content in milk in all animals, especially dairy cows), black treacle or molasses, honey, raw eggs, linseed tea, calamus root, pine kernels, melilot, lucerne (blue or yellow) milk-wort (whole plant), dill seed, slippery-elm flour, marshmallow root (the three latter all obtainable in tree-barks'-blend flour), finely cut borage leaves mixed in with the milk, also sprinkled on the meat, and, lastly, an abundance of good drinking water.

The gun-dog expert Mrs M.K. Wentworth-Smith (of the Yelme Golden Retrievers, Thetford, Norfolk, England) and her kennel manageress (Miss Eva B. Todd) have sent me a very comprehensive and interesting report on the effects of herbal medicine and natural rearing on the Yelme brood bitches.

After many years of rigid adherence to natural feeding, combined with herbal additions, I am more than delighted with the result.

In the case of in-whelp and nursing bitches the difference is most marked. The bitches retain their full health, spirits, and activity (as far as this latter is possible), produce their puppies with no distress, even if it is a first litter at five years old. Lactation is good, the bitches are willing, nay, anxious, to suckle their puppies so long as a drop of milk remains – the flow usually continuing abundant for at least *ten to twelve weeks*. Then, without exception, they follow

Nature's design in vomiting up for their litter the food necessary to follow the milk diet. In fact, it is difficult to persuade them to renounce their maternal cares at all.

During this period our experience is that the bitches retain their own well-being and vitality and are still well covered instead of having that 'pulled-down' look, nor do they lose their dark pigmentation; in fact, this is even more marked.

This method, by following the full cycle of Nature's design, also appears to ensure the brood bitch regaining her pre-birth neat and elegant figure – no unsightly or vulnerable 'under-carriage' remaining to destroy symmetry, reduce activity, and get torn or injured when at field work.

Medicines A healthy bitch does not require medicines, especially not the general concoctions of the chemist. But Nature herself has provided a few plants which are of use in helping milk flow – marshmallow plant, flowers or leaves, is highly recommended for increasing the milk flow, so also are fennel herb, seeds or leaves, and borage, already described. Grated raw carrot given on the meat feed is also excellent and raw chopped dates given with the cereal feed. Raw eggs – but not more than three per week – are beneficial for this purpose. The milk flow can be used as an anti-worm aid for the suckling puppies if garlic is fed to the bitch daily throughout the nursing period. The penetrative powers of garlic are well known and well proved. The volatile oils of the garlic plant possess the unique powers of entering almost every cell of the body, but especially the body fluids, blood, urine, and, in the case of the female, the milk flow. It is well known what great care farmers take to keep their milking cows away from all contact with the garlic plant. I was intrigued to read in Thomas Hardy's great novel, *Tess of the D'Urbervilles* – which, incidentally, is a masterpiece of country-life description – how all the milkmaids are detailed to search the meadows for a few garlic plants which had entered and rooted in the meadow, and which were flavouring the milk yield of the entire herd of a hundred or more cattle – so powerful is the garlic plant's power of milk-flow penetration, and so equally powerful the kine's natural desire to partake of the wonderfully medicinal herb whenever the plant grows within reach. Garlic dosage will serve the additional purpose of helping to keep the bitch herself worm free during the vital time of the nursing and, later, the weaning of her puppies, and can help the pups through the milk.

DISTEMPER (see Chapter 7) An in-whelp bitch that develops distemper, treated by internal-cleansing method, can whelp a perfectly normal litter. I have nursed many in-whelp bitches through distemper for breeders, and have seen excellent litters with no sign at all of their mother's disease.

ECLAMPSIA The bitch may sometimes suffer from a glandular disturbance generally known as eclampsia. The theory much in vogue with dog breeders is that this disorder (a form of epileptic fits or severe total body cramp) is caused solely by calcium deficiency in the blood, a sudden drainage of her calcium. The mineral which is actually lacking in most cases is iodine; the only healthful way of supplying this in its natural organic form is in the cells of most seaweeds and some vegetables. The giving of chemical iodine is unnatural and very harmful. In the rarer cases, when it is indeed calcium drainage, hypodermic injection of calcium into the bloodstream is the quickest cure. Neglected eclampsia can cause death.

FEVER Fever of the puerperal type is not common in bitches. But if a case should occur, then immediate strong dosing with herbal antiseptic tablets is required, and fasting on honey-water. Give a nightly laxative, of senna pods preferably. The litter must be removed from the dam, and hand fed. The dam's milk must be expressed by hand three times daily. When the fever subsides and the bitch is back on a solid-foods diet, her puppies can be restored.

MASTITIS This condition is not very common in the canine race for, unlike the domestic cow or goat, the bitch is allowed to suckle her offspring as nature intended, and is not subjected to milking machines, and so forth. The ailment is most commonly caused by feeble puppies who are unable to suckle their dam strongly and therefore do not empty the breasts several times daily. Congestion results and mastitis develops. The typical symptom is swelling and hardness of the whole milk-secreting area, and often a few degrees of fever. The bitch usually refuses to allow the puppies to feed from her because of the pain caused by the congestion.

Treatment The puppies should be removed from the bitch and, meantime, hand reared. The milk glands must be emptied of all milk by hand expression, first applying cloths dipped in hot sage water to the breasts. This should be carried out four to five times during the day. The milk-glands area should be bathed with a brew of elder and dock leaves – one handful of each brewed in 1½ pints of water. Internal treatment is one day's complete fast on water only, with four herbal antiseptic tablets given twice daily (average breed); a laxative in the evening, then a fluid diet of milk and honey for several days until normality is restored. The puppies can then feed again from their dam. This treatment, which I originated for cows and goats, gave very good results for these animals and was much recommended by that great farmer, Sir Albert Howard.

GENERAL TREATMENT OF THE BROOD BITCH

A brood bitch requires careful treatment, both psychological and practical. General treatment not only affects the bitch's own health but, further, has an important bearing upon the health of the litter, both before and after birth. I will deal first with the psychological handling.

I absolutely deplore the turning of any animal into a mere breeding machine, but especially so the dog, because of its great capacity for affection towards its human owners, and its great gifts of intelligence, both practical and spiritual. Throughout England there are dozens of kennels that keep their bitches virtually prisoners: year after year they are brought out of prison confinement for mating and whelping, and then sent back again to the long months of mental boredom, their world of no larger interest than that of a wooden kennel and a concrete run (for persons who keep their dogs as kennel prisoners usually favour the concrete run: it is simpler to keep 'clean' than the more healthful brick or natural grass run). It is no wonder, following such treatment, that the offspring of pedigree stock have acquired the popular reputation of being 'idiots'. In my eyes the brood bitch should be looked upon as a highly important, and therefore privileged, person. This is only rightful when it is appreciated that the future continuance of any particular strain of dog is greatly dependent upon the health and the breeding powers of the brood bitch.

Dr Jane Goodall, famous for her work with chimpanzees and who is a foremost worker on wild-life research, education and conservation, mentioned in a recent broadcast for the BBC the sad problem of chimpanzees in captivity, the problem of boredom.

Like all creatures (including the dog and cat), chimpanzees want to work. They also want to be kept amused, not shut away in enforced inactivity. Think again, and I stress this, of the caged laboratory dogs and cats. The only interruption in their day and night of total isolation is the visit of their tormentors to give them their daily doses of *pain*. Dr Goodall stated that long sessions of boredom can cause character changes and health decline in chimpanzees.

She also told of the passion for honey (and mustard!) observed in chimpanzees. Both foods are excellent for all creatures. Honey is enjoyed not merely by man, but by all living things from donkey to bird – even plants like honey! Only let honey be pure, not cheated by man by the adding of white sugar, feeding this harmful substance to the bees themselves for the making of 'quick' honey not derived from flower nectar, or mixing sugar into the honey itself. Honey does great good to body and mind, and that is why it is mentioned in relation to boredom because dogs shut away for long hours in isolation can be rewarded by some spoonfuls of honey. Anticipation of reward can ease the mental pain of boredom.

Throughout the in-whelp period the bitch requires increased human companionship and an extra amount of exercise, so that she is kept mentally alert and active. A feeling of absolute trust must be developed between owner and bitch, so that in the case of any whelping complications arising the bitch will yield her body with an absolutely calm mind to the care of the human owner (this factor is of tremendous importance in the saving of a bitch and her litter in freak or complicated whelpings). Also such relationship removes all risks of a bitch savaging her puppies, which event in almost every case – and it is common enough in general dog breeding – is purely a matter of nervous hysteria. The bitch should be given all protection from alarming noises when with her litter, and she should never be compelled to soil her bed. I have known kennel owners with nursing bitches leave their kennels for a full day while attending dog shows, leaving bitches confined with their litters in closed kennels. Such absolute cruelty appears to be quite habitual in general dog breeding. Is it then to be wondered at that many bitches savage their puppies?

Practical treatment is dependent on correct diet, as already described, and frequent, regular, and abundant daily exercise. For the first few days, of course, very little exercise is required, but the bitch must be allowed away from her litter at frequent intervals in order to stretch her limbs, pass urine, and cleanse her bowels. Also at such times her lungs are panting for abundant draughts of fresh out-of-doors air. Regular daily grooming is also an essential, both to keep her body clean and to assist complete circulation of the blood; thorough daily grooming is also very beneficial to the nervous system. To assist general body cleansing, the fasting treatment is also to be utilized. A regular weekly half-day fast is sufficient, with one whole day per month. The one whole day per month, both during the in-whelp period and the nursing period, is *essential* to true total health and must not be neglected.

It is natural for the in-whelp bitch to fast on the day she is due to whelp and for at least twenty-four hours following whelping. Cats will often refuse all food for two or three days after they have given birth to their kittens.

Domestication has changed this and altered natural instincts. The body has no time or forces to expend on food digestion during the important time of birth, nor immediately following birth when the temporarily weakened system requires strengthening, not through unwanted heavy foods, but through rest, sleep, and absolute quiet.

At the most, brood bitches can be fed milk and honey on the day due to whelp, and very watered milk and honey during the day following whelping. Then slowly introduce cereal feeds and milk. Do not give a heavy meal of meat until the third day after whelping. In cases of exhaustion, fresh grape juice (or, if not available, then bottled grape juice) can be given as a medicine every two hours or so. An average amount would be two tablespoons for a medium size bitch. Give also honey.

When whelping is prolonged in the case of big litters, one puppy only should be left with the mother while she is whelping; the others, after cleaning by the dam, should be placed apart on a warm bottle covered by a blanket from contact with the puppies, to await the arrival of all the litter.

Leaving puppies under the mother when whelping may cause fatalities. In the wild the death of several puppies is probably accounted for by Nature; in professional breeding the best of the litter may be lost accidently this way.

DRYING OFF MILK

Unlike the milch animals, such as the farm cow and goat who have unnatural, large development of the udder, the bitch usually loses her milk easily when her litter is weaned at nine weeks or twelve. But in the rare cases of prolonged milk, or the troublesome milk which comes in false pregnancies, milk can be dried up by internal and external treatments with herbs.

Internally give three times daily, strong draughts of common garden mint, made into a tea, or the great reed, *Arundo donax*, given internally: macerate and give two teaspoons twice daily. Or raw cucumber juice can be given also, two dessertspoons morning and night. Externally apply camphorated oil by patting gently into the breasts (not by rubbing). Have the oil fairly hot, and apply morning and night for one week. Then follow on treatment with warm vinegar in place of the camphorated oil.

PROTECTION OF THE BITCH ON HEAT

I have never been troubled with many unwanted dogs around my premises when my Afghan bitches are on heat. I take careful precautions that dogs do not find my bitches. The following is my method: for the three weeks of being on heat the bitch is only exercised on the leash. Wherever she urinates or excretes, a mixture of stove paraffin and water (two of paraffin to one of water) is poured on the place. This breaks her scent. The mixture is carried in a bottle when out at exercise. Alternative protection (and harmless to the ground) is the use of a pungent powder, such as talcum powder of strong scent or NR herbal protection powder containing wormwood herb of intense bitterness. The powders can be eked out cheaply with wood ash. In addition, apply a few drops of oil of eucalyptus on the bitch's hind-quarters, diluted by putting on to a piece of cold-water-dampened cotton wool. Do not let this touch the bare skin of the vagina or anus. If despite this disguise of scent, the one odd dog finds that the bitch is on heat, he gets such a bad reception with flung plant-pots and buckets of water that he soon finds it is not worthwhile to continue his unwelcome visits! When a car is available, then simply exercise the bitch far from home premises, and merely sprinkle the disguise thing or things around the gate outside.

SPAYING OF BITCHES The mystic poet and prophet, Percy Bysshe Shelley, wrote that man's dominance over the animals is one of disease and pain for the animals. Too often this is true. Spaying of bitches is total in selfishness. The whole life of the animal is dedicated to procreation. If breeding is prevented, then the heart has gone out of life, and likewise the survival on earth through the children. Spaying also destroys the whole natural rhythm of the body and the spayed animal becomes sluggish in both body and mind, and is simply a creature left half alive. The same applies to the castrating of male animals. Spaying is only permissible when it has been proved that further offspring would endanger the life of the mother.

My recent booklet entitled *Against the Castrating and Spaying of Dogs (and Cats)* gives much more information on this subject.

3

Care of Puppies in the Nest

Very little attention to suckling puppies is required, from the time of birth until the commencement of weaning in the fourth week or so. If the bitch is in normal health, she will keep the puppies clean, warm, and well nourished without any human interference. Indeed, the more the bitch is left in quiet solitude, the better it is for the litter. It is the bitch only who requires attention, and such care has been described in the preceding chapter.

The docking of tails and the removal of dew-claws in the chosen breeds should be carried out as early as possible, around the third day in healthy puppies, if they *must* be done: I hate tail docking. The wounds must not be dressed with iodine or any chemical disinfectant, most of which retard healing and are the frequent cause of puppy losses at such times. Use preferably witch hazel extract diluted, which is purely herbal – one teaspoon witch hazel to two teaspoons water – or a herbal brew made from elder-tree leaves, or blackberry leaves, or whole sprigs of rosemary or rue. To make the herbal brew: finely shred two tablespoons of freshly gathered, preferably, or dry leaves or flowering sprigs of the above-mentioned herbs, scald with ½ pint of boiling water, allow to brew overnight, then strain and use cold. Thoroughly bathe the wounded areas with the herbal brew. The same antiseptic herbal treatment can be applied to the umbilical area of the pups.

Puppies in the nest should be kept in the semi-dark until their eyes have opened. The building housing them must be absolutely clean and well ventilated. Dirty kennels are the cause of the loss of far more newly born puppies than ever die from disease. Breeders habitually keep litters in much-used kennels, where the wooden boards are urine-soaked and worm- and various bacteria-impregnated. Kennels used for puppy-rearing purposes *must* be regularly long-term rested and whitewashed. To put successive litters into the same kennels is simply inviting general disease development. A clean, rested, newly whitewashed kennel must be used for each litter reared. Blankets as bedding should be avoided; newspaper is far better.

HAND REARING This is an unnatural process and really should have no place in this book on natural rearing. Every bitch should be able to rear her own litter without human interference. However, breeders at various times have had to hand-rear an odd litter, and Natural Rearing principles of diet have been applied with great success. Indeed, bench champions have been produced from such rearings.

It is impossible to give rules for feeding times. The new-born puppies being suckled by their dam feed whenever hungry and sleep away the rest of the time. But feeds should be very frequent for the first weeks: two-hourly by day and four-hourly by night. Then go on to three-hourly by day and only once in the night, but begin the new day's feeds at dawn, eventually decreasing to four-hourly by day, no night feed, but starting as before at dawn. Diet should be natural foods, raw cow or goat milk diluted with water from flaked oats which have been soaked overnight, and honey added. To every cup of milk add two dessertspoons oats water, one small teaspoon of honey and a few drops of almond, corn or sesame oil; add egg yolk, but only twice a day and not every day. The oil is needed because the milk of bitches is richer in fats than cow or goat milk. Do not use sheep's milk – it is over-fatty for infant puppies. This mixture should be given tepid – do not spoil the milk by overheating it; but do not give cold food to infant puppies. Chamomile herb tea is soothing: use it for soaking the oat flakes. Use a small feeding-bottle with a finely pierced rubber teat. In the second week, NR tree-barks' gruel can be added to the milk for extra soothing power and for increased vitamins and minerals. Numerous animals of many kinds have been hand-reared on this food. Not only puppies and kittens, but also goat kids, lambs, young owls and hawks – all achieved great health on bottle-fed feeds of goat's milk and tree-barks' (slippery-elm, etc) flour. A mere pinch of this flour per puppy, at first, increasing to a half and then a whole teaspoon as the puppies grow on. They should also be fed drinks of barley water, several times daily, for its slightly laxative and further soothing properties. This should be made by pouring hot (not boiled) water over whole-grain barley, allowing this to stand over-night, and then expressing the liquid through a piece of muslin.

New-born puppies must be kept warm with the aid of a well-blanketed hot-water bottle. Their anal and bladder areas should be kept clean with cotton wool swabs dipped into warm water, squeezed semi-dry, and then a little olive oil applied; a good talcum powder is also useful. Clean the puppies after every feed. At a very early age puppies should have access to shallow dishes of water. In the wilds they lick at dew-wet herbage and get water that way. Puppies hand-reared by this method seldom scour, do not develop pot-bellies, and are very active and contented. Only occasionally will a bottle-feeding puppy, not carefully watched, eat to a state of severe bloating. This pressure of excess food must be removed immediately. Insert a leafy stem of any plant into the anus and gently press with the hands on the stomach; this will cause the puppy to evacuate and the swollen body will deflate. Let the puppy miss the next meal to rest its stomach.

Finally, a loud-ticking alarm clock wrapped in a warm cloth gives the puppies the impression that their mother is with them, and they nestle around this.

At the age of one month, if weather permits, the rule should be outdoors by day and indoors when the sun goes down. A wooden packing case, or a Bedouin-type tent made of sacks stretched over a wire frame, provides shelter from wind. The puppy's own body heat will soon warm up such places. Puppies love to sun themselves, but some shade should always be available so they can get out of the sun when they want to. I hate the rearing of puppies indoors in stuffy rooms.

I recently hand-reared a litter of Afghans when the dam was poisoned. This litter produced Turkuman Nissim's Sea-Lavender, a fawn-grey male who for a long time was the unbeaten running champion among the Afghans and salukis of all Israel (competing with the famed racing Bedouin salukis of the Negev and Sinai deserts). My own dog from this same hand-reared litter, Turkuman Nissim's Sea-Campion, a black, is so strong that I require two leashes to hold him when he sees cats he wishes to chase. He has not yet been to the Windhound Club races to challenge his famous racing brother, but at his first show he was made Best of Breed by USA hound expert Lee Abraham, who commented in the show ring that she had seldom seen such muscular development and pure *strength* in any hound. His son, Turkuman Güzel Laurel-leaves of Queen of Sheba's House, also a black, later won all the Afghan hound races in Israel, beating his uncle, Sea-Lavender.

AILMENTS OF THE NEW-BORN LITTER

Puppies in the nest generally remain immune from the major ailments such as distemper, nervous diseases, and other ailments of the adult dog. The principal disorders of early puppyhood are: 'fading' disease, now usually attributed to beta haemolytic streptococcal disease (b.h.s.), although sometimes this may be brought on by a toxic or very acid milk flow of the dam; dysentery, or scouring, worm infestation – especially by wire-worms, which can frequently kill off very young puppies – skin disorders, especially mange. For detailed curative treatments, readers are referred to Part Two of this book where the ailments are separately and fully dealt with, both preventative and curative treatments being given. In Part Two there is an especially large section on streptococcal disease. For cure of this now very common canine ailment, my internal cleansing herbal treatment has been immensely successful, having overcome the disease in many of Europe's famous kennels. And newly, since the 1980s, there is the very serious ailment of virus type, parvovirus.

COCCIDIOSIS   Sera and chemical drug treatments completely failed to cure streptococcal disease. There has had to be found some scapegoat for the failure of the expensive orthodox treatments inflicted on the harassed dog breeders. When unnatural treatments have failed to cure the streptococcal infection – indeed, in many cases have aggravated the trouble – some reason must be forthcoming for the failure; and now, therefore, breeders are being told that there is yet a new canine ailment responsible for barren bitches or fading out of litters: this is *Coccidiosis*. Cocci are single spherical-shaped bacteria (in contrast to the streptococci bacteria which are found in chains); just as with streptococci, they are very common, and are very widely distributed; they can, likewise, be found in perfectly healthy body tissue. Coccidiosis has long been a bugbear in goat, rabbit, and poultry breeding, but hitherto it has not been given much publicity in canine medicine, streptococcal disease dominating the stage. I advise all intelligent dog breeders to treat this ailment in the exact way that they are treating b.h.s. Remove the root cause of the disease by replacing unnatural rearing methods by natural ones, and by treating the actual ailment entirely on the system advocated for streptococcal disease, which treatment has been so unfailingly successful. Professor M. Perek, DVM, of the Agricultural Faculty of the Hebrew University, Jerusalem, told me that one of his workers demonstrated that coccidiosis in poultry could be cured with the use of garlic given to the infected birds.

DYSENTERY (DIARRHOEA, SCOURING) Sometimes very young puppies, perhaps under one week of age, begin scouring – usually a grey or pale yellow diarrhoea. Unless this trouble is checked the puppies will die. General treatment is: remove the litter from the dam for two days, give six small meals per day (hand rearing) of very diluted tepid water and honey: about one-quarter teaspoonful of honey to one dessertspoonful tepid (unboiled) water, at each meal, average size breeds. Give one leaf-extract tablet (now called Herbal Compound), cut into smaller pieces, average size breed. Bigger doses for older puppies. Or give a tea of bilberry leaves. Then after two days, return litter to the dam, who herself should have been fasted for at least one day and dosed with leaf-extract tablets – treatment of the dam being followed as a precautionary measure in case it is her milk which is causing the litter to scour. Needless to say, the litter must be kept very warm throughout the time of the removal from the dam, using flannel-covered hot-water bottles; and they must be kept clean with olive oil applied on cotton wool with talcum powder used in order to prevent skin chafing and soreness. If the scouring returns, then the treatment must be repeated at short intervals. This treatment has saved hundreds of very sick litters, and puppies so treated have grown into healthy ones, speedily.

In prolonged dysentery, dehydration must be prevented: it is always dangerous to life. Give anti-dehydration mixture – a level teaspoon each of honey and glucose, a small half teaspoon (or less) of table salt, to make a small cup of liquid by adding barley water (home made) (see Parvovirus, p. 226).

The litter should be weaned strictly on tree-barks' food flour, which has stomachic and intestinal healing properties.

'FADING OUT' of young puppies. This trouble is fully dealt with under the Streptococcal disease section, p. 252. At the present time, hepatitis is largely blamed for puppy losses. General treatment is through the dam, prenatal and post-natal. The following report is of interest, from Mrs Winifred Barber, journalist and judge, writing in *Our Dogs*, Scottish terrier breed notes.

Miss Gwen Southwell reports: 'I read your notes a few weeks ago about bitches missing, etc, and there has been a lot of talk about puppies fading out, so I thought I would tell you of my experience with my winning Fox Terrier bitch, Fulgents Nigella. I have for some time been interested in herbal remedies, and about six weeks before she had her litter I gave her one leaf-extract tablet a day. She had four dogs and one bitch, all sturdy, lovely puppies, yet they seemed a bit discontented, although they fed well. On the fourth day one of the dogs became distended and very uncomfortable . . . [A typical condition of 'fading out' – J. de B.L.] I thought that he was going to become a 'wailer' and that I should lose him – it used to be quite a common thing for me to lose one in this way before the war. However, I gave the mother four leaf-extract tablets (they are wonderful for any sign of strep.), and two garlic herbal tablets a day, and next day the puppy was normal and all have gone on very well since . . . the dam continued to have a herbal tablet every day. Since weaning, the puppies have had a ten-day course, and I haven't seen a sign of a worm from them. My puppies always had lots in the old days. I am so pleased to have saved my puppy. I hope that my experience may be of use to others; it is so disappointing when they fade out.

PUPPY SKIN RASH   This skin rash is not to be confused with follicular mange, with which skin ailment many puppies are born, coming into life already infected from the dam; this follicular condition is quite often found in smooth-haired dachshunds, litters being born totally devoid of hair. In such cases the skin has a blue-grey hue and is sweaty to the feel and is also evil-smelling. This is totally different from the rash which sometimes affects unweaned puppies, bred from a bitch that is not in normal health. The skin ailment is often called 'milk-rash' and is typified by crusty scabs covering large areas, sometimes the entire body. The body hair is not generally lost. Treatment is internal with leaf extract, average one crushed tablet per puppy per day, plus external bathing of the body surface with cotton-wool swabs dipped into a brew of blackberry leaves. The blackberry lotion is wonderfully effective in treatment of all eczematous conditions. Clover flowers, and/or leaves, or elder blossom can be added to the brew with much benefit.

WORM INFESTATION   Worm infestation in newly born puppies is a fatal condition and often results in early death, especially if the worms are of the wire variety. This trouble would never happen if the dam received proper prenatal treatment and was in sound health at the time of whelping. But it is freely acknowledged that the ova of worms can circulate in the bloodstream of the dam and thus reach the bodies of the unborn puppies, so that the litter is infested before birth. Treatment must be carried out first through the dam, who should be dosed with herbal worm tablets. In severe infestation of puppies, give them one tablet (average dose) cut up small, then follow the worm tablets, fifteen minutes later, with a dessertspoon dose of Milk of Magnesia, which has use as a mild laxative, but I do not advise as an antacid in canine use. Or senna laxative can be given: one large pod soaked in one dessertspoon of cold water for approximately four hours; a pinch of powdered ginger should be added to this. This is for one puppy.

I must here stress that there is no advantage at all in blasting out by means of various chemicals (bowel irritants mostly) vast numbers of worms; the injury thus caused is twice that which the worms themselves are able to cause, worms in general feeding on the mucus and other impurities accumulated in the intestines. The aim should be to remove those impurities on which the worms are feeding and in which they have embedded themselves. Remove the impurities first by the aid of that proved internal herbal cleanser, garlic, rue, etc, via the mother's milk, and then by a laxative and restorative weaning diet – especially a diet of whole raw foods.

WEANING

It is impossible to give strict rules for puppy weaning, as weaning differs greatly with individual puppies. But I can say with authority that hurried weaning, careless weaning, unnatural weaning, can ruin a puppy's health so that ever afterwards there is a predisposition to fits, hysteria, gastritis, worm infestation. It is worth taking all possible care. It is a matter of true personal breeding skill to know what exact quantities of food to feed to individual puppies, also when to feed and when to fast – for fasting should play an important part in all animal rearing, although that measure is usually totally ignored by the majority of breeders.

On one subject, however, it is possible to speak very precisely, and that is concerning the correct time for weaning. One of the greatest errors of Western dog weaning (and also child weaning) is the general haste to get the puppies to partake of solid food. In dog breeding the great incentive appears to be commercial, i.e. the earlier the weaning, the earlier the puppies can be offered for sale. Slow weaning as opposed to hasty weaning is a necessity, because Nature has not prepared the intestines and stomachs of infant carnivores for the digestion of anything other than milk food until or after the fourth week. Food – especially the usual starchy white-flour puppy-weaning foods fed to the puppy before the fourth week – will be digested to some extent, but at the same time it is distending the stomach and intestines and creating acid condition of the bloodstream and a sour mucus-laden condition of the digestive organs, thus making an ideal state for the development of worm ova, streptococcal bacteria, and distemper disease. Wean the puppies in their fourth week on raw goat or cow milk thickened with honey. Milk should be fed tepid-to-cold, never hot. Then for extra feeding value, strengthen the milk with a preparation of slippery-elm tree-barks' flour, making sure that the slippery elm is pure and unrefined. Slippery elm is not a cheap substance, and consequently some manufacturers of this food, wanting to make the high profits common to commercial foods, add such quantities of cheap white flour to the elm that the food becomes nothing more than flour flecked with particles of elm bark. The genuine preparation, as I sell it, is a brown colour with a very strong, characteristic smell.

I once met a well-known North England breeder of wire fox terriers, who was a long-time sufferer from gastric disease, and on his doctor's advice was on a diet of milk and slippery-elm food. He had made no progress in curing his ailment. I asked him to send me a sample of the elm food which he was taking. I saw that the food was a useless commercial product, elm flour adulterated beyond chance of possessing any curative properties. I therefore sent a supply of the genuine, natural product, and the improvement in the man's health was instant and remarkable, gastric pain disappeared and he began to feel marvellously well. I am relating this now to point out the importance of ascertaining that foods used are in a natural state as opposed to the general over-refined or adulterated products wherein the natural properties of the ingredients are almost totally removed during manufacture. The reasons for interference with natural foods are manifold. To enhance the keeping properties of food is a very usual reason – in short, to enable the selling of stale products; or to lower the manufacturers' own production costs and to increase their trade profits. For instance, in the processing of natural wheat grain, big side profits are to be made from the sale of the bran and of the wheat germ – the extraction of the vital 'life' of the wheat in its germ also enhances the long-term keeping properties of the resultant flours, important for profitable commerce.

Mention should here and now be made of that other commonly spoiled, vitally important, puppy-weaning food – milk. For milk to be true food, it should be raw, unheated fluid food from healthy goats or cows. The sterilizing of milk in pasteurization, and likewise the drying of milk to turn it into powder form, both destroy the vital vitamin and cosmic properties which are so peculiar to milk and are so very delicate therein. The milk of herbivorous animals is – or should be – mainly the vitamin-rich herbage and vegetable matter on which the animal has been feeding, in general liquid suspension. (Note how quickly and surely such high-tasting foods as garlic, various root vegetables, and other plants – the milk of clover-fed cattle is honey-sweet to the taste – enter the milk flow.) All leaf matter contains vital forces other than vitamins. Professor Dr Szekely describes these forces as 'cosmic'; they come to the plant from the radiations from sun, moon, and stars; the forces contain great restorative, regenerative, and healing powers; in raw, natural, untreated milk most of these forces – so vital to health – are found intact. There is no substitute for clean, raw milk. I appreciate that such food is difficult to obtain at present, as in the modern, ugly commercial farming called 'intensive' milch animals are often confined in enclosures and do not graze pastures at all. But if people want to breed dogs they should make adequate preparations for the proper feeding of them; they should keep goats. For instance, who but an idiot would attempt to rear a horse without having any grazing ground available for the animal? And yet hundreds of breeders mate their bitches and proceed to rear a litter without having made any provision for the supplying of those foodstuffs vital to true and normal health. No wonder that puppy losses are so prevalent nowadays, and subhealth is the general rule among most pedigree dogs rather than the exception.

The following opinion on milk as a food will uphold my own findings on the subject. From Dr John Harvey Kellogg's treatise, *Auto-Intoxication*:

Milk is a sort of fluid tissue and like other tissues is prepared from the blood; hence it is not surprising that the profound scientific study to which this remarkable food substance has been subjected within recent years has brought to light the fact that milk possesses some of the properties of the living blood from which it is produced. While still warm with animal heat *freshly drawn milk, like the blood, possesses the power to combat and destroy germs.* Milk contains various antibodies which are found in the blood, agglutins, anti-toxins, and opsonins. It must be admitted that these last-named elements of milk have been so recently discovered that their relation and value to human life and health are not yet fully understood.

A HOME-MADE SUPER HEALTH PUPPY FOOD   Powdered barley flakes (grind barley flakes through a handmill) a half cupful. Add to this the following: a heaped teaspoon of powdered slippery (red) elm bark. This is a beige powder, very aromatic, makes a jelly when mixed with water. One teaspoon powdered almonds. Half teaspoon crushed anise seeds.

Mix well. Then make into a paste with a heaped teaspoon of honey. Then add an approximate tablespoon of hottish water (not too hot to kill the life in the honey) to bind the mixture together. Finally, stir in slowly one cupful of warm milk (not Long-life type of milk). Repeat this meal twice daily. Also give some to the mother of the pups.

As the puppies approach their fifth week the milk food should be thickened with whole-grain flaked cereals, making a beginning with flaked barley, which is the most simple cereal from a digestive point of view. If not obtainable, use flaked oats. Soon the first teeth will be felt in the gums. Now add also a good gruel made with milk.

Now at this time, towards the fifth week, raw meat should be introduced. The natural instinct of the bitch when in the wild state (and common to all carnivores) is to semi-digest flesh food in her own stomach, and then to vomit up the food for the use of her whelps. Therefore, keeping this in mind, it should be understood that some preparation of the meat will be necessary. Early preparation of meat is simply the rendering of it in as easily digestible form as possible, by means *other than* cooking. The meat should be hung for some time before use in order to soften it, and only lean meat should be fed at first. A big slice should be selected and the surface then scraped with a knife, the soft red flesh which then adheres to the blade of the knife or the edge of the spoon (a spoon can be used for meat scraping) should then be removed and fed to the puppy in bulk. Ration for a first meal for an average size puppy would be approximately one teaspoon. This quantity should be increased every three days, until, at eight weeks of age, the puppy (average size breed) is having two tablespoons of finely shredded meat twice per day. By that time – eight weeks – the puppy will be fully weaned. The future diet of the growing puppy up to adult age has already been given in the Diets at the end of Chapter 1. Do not mince the meat.

Remember that every ounce, every particle of food contributes to the strength of puppy limbs, therefore let every meal given be of maximum health in natural concentration and preparation.

A properly weaned puppy is a joy to see and possess. It has come into the world with a set of 'brand-new' organs: heart, brain, liver, kidneys, etc. All are new, clean, unspoiled. It is each puppy's right that it be fed foods which will not damage or degenerate its new body, but improve and safeguard its health, so that it will never know the pain and distress of worm infestation, rickets, scouring, skin eruptions. The great naturalist, W.H. Hudson, said of that natural-living race, the gypsies (before inroads of civilization and faulty modern diet caused the health degeneration which has become prevalent among them today): 'I've never seen a gypsy with a cold, a headache, indigestion or backache. Wind, snow, rain, they maintain their splendid health.' I can say the same of a truly naturally reared puppy: I've never seen a sickly one or a weakly one; they flourish from the day of birth and are weaned as stalwart, independent little individuals, ready to play their important parts in the canine world.

Cleanliness is a first essential. The puppies should be cleanly housed, and bedded on good quality hay or straw (preferably hay). For although hay bedding is supposed to encourage vermin, there are health-giving properties in the dry produce of green meadows not possessed by any other form of bedding; and in any case the firm skins and 'tough' body hair of really healthy puppies do not encourage insect parasites to linger there. Such vermin go farther afield for the weak-tissued, unhealthy skins of animals degenerate in health, for under such circumstances they can take a firm foothold from which they will not easily be dislodged until the death of the animal host. The persistence with which fleas and lice return again and again to the bodies of unhealthy animals, as soon as chemical warfare upon the skin vermin is relaxed by the breeder, has always impressed me. The growing puppies must have daily access to grassland. The dew which forms on clean, healthy grass – barren, sour grass lacks dew formation – is an important tonic for young puppies, and most puppies which have not totally lost their natural instincts will be found licking eagerly at the surface of dew or rain-wet herbage. The puppies' search for moisture indicates that a feed of water must be made available as soon as their eyes open. Water should always be present in the kennel run (not in the kennel, except with in-whelp bitches, which frequently require to partake of water during the night), other than shortly before or after meals. The partaking of water while food digestion is in progress both washes the food over quickly from the stomach down into the intestines and dilutes the digestive juices.

Sleep is as important to growing puppies as is good natural food. Young puppies should be put to sleep in well-ventilated kennels for several hours at a fixed hour during every day. They should also be put to bed early and given the great benefit of early rising. No breeder who is himself a late riser, and who habitually deprives his dogs of the benefits of the sweet vital air of the early-morning hours, will ever make a true success of dog rearing. As a university student, I acquired the bad habit of late-night study and consequent late-morning rising; it was dog ownership and the necessity of giving them the essential morning exercise which caused me to return to natural hours in keeping with the true laws of Nature. I love the early mornings, and nothing will ever again deprive me of them.

Puppies not not require sunlight on their bodies before their eyes are opened at their tenth to fourteenth day, and even afterwards they should be shaded from very strong sunlight until their newly opened eyes have strengthened. Very young puppies will scream lustily if exposed to very strong sunlight without any access to shade. When it is remembered that in the wild state they were sheltered in dark caves during the first weeks of their lives, the dislike of the very young puppy for sunlight can be understood. But as soon as the puppies have reached the weaning stage, and their limbs have become active, then sunlight is one of the most important attributes to successful rearing. Indeed, it is an essential: as with a growing plant, no creature, apart from the nocturnal ones – and they bask in moonlight – can flourish when kept in the dark; sun is the supreme life-giver, for without sun there can be no life.

Puppies, from their early weeks, should be given separate dishes when weaned. Be strict concerning this, as competitive feeding causes overeating and thus digestive ailments. It is natural in the wild for each fox or wolf cub to run off with its portion of torn flesh and devour this at safe distance from the other cubs. Only by separate feeding can the owner be sure that each puppy receives its proper share of food.

4
Care of Cats

Hitherto I have not included cats in any of my veterinary herbal books, except in passing or to indicate where diet or treatment was similar to dogs. I added this chapter and further information about the domestic cat to the fifth edition of this book, giving it its new title of *The Complete Herbal Handbook for the Dog and Cat* and, some years ago, I added a chapter on farm cats for the Dutch edition of my *Complete Herbal Handbook for Farm and Stable*. In 1991 my completely new book *Cats Naturally: Natural Rearing for Healthier Cats* was published by Faber.

It is true to say that all veterinary herbal treatments are applicable to all creatures – from the bee to the camel, for example. In fact, a chapter on herbal treatment for bees is included in the farm and stable handbook, and I successfully treated with herbs many ailing Bedouin camels when I was living in various parts of North Africa and the Middle East.

In all editions of my canine herbal I have emphasized that all treatments of ailments for dogs are equally appropriate for cats.

In that excellent and highly informative veterinary book – *Complete Guide to Natural Health for Dogs and Cats* by Richard H. Pitcairn, DVM, PhD and Susan Hubble Pitcairn (Rodale Press, USA) – Dr Pitcairn lists some recommended books which have relation to the natural care of these animals.

His view of my book is: 'A classic on the subject. Valuable

information and anecdote on herbal therapy, natural feeding and health care. Orientated towards dogs, *but much of it is adaptable to cats.*' (My italics.)

Readers who want to adapt canine veterinary herbal treatments to cats have merely to refer to the canine ailments which are similar to the feline: almost every canine ailment has its feline counterpart. That true scourge, the modern canine virus disease – parvovirus – is, for instance, so similar in symptoms to one of the worst of the feline ailments, feline panleukopenia, that vets are commonly using the general feline vaccine for that disease – not that I approve of this: results have not been impressive, but the disease symptoms are highly similar.

Hepatitis treatment is identical for dogs and cats, as it is for humans, and the same treatments are applicable for ailments of lungs, kidneys and nerves, external for skin ailments, including ringworm and the troublesome ticks, lice and fleas, and internal for parasites of the worms class, especially tapeworm so prevalent in the modern cat.

Indeed the only real difference in herbal treatment to be made between dogs and cats is in the matter of dosage, the cat requiring far smaller dosage than the dog of average size breed. For example, the cat would do well on the small dosage advised for the toy breeds of dog.

In any case, some overdosage would not do any harm because I prescribe only the harmless herbs in my books and articles and lectures and deliberately avoid the poisonous ones. These are never needed and there is always an alternative safe herb to do the same work as the poisonous one.

What the cat does need and does deserve is its own special diet.

Many years ago I had some feline diets printed for private use among cat lovers known to me personally, but for this new book I have now revised the cat diet very fully, bringing it right up to date with my findings in modern natural nutrition. Many cat owners, on my advice, have had their cats on Natural Rearing for many years and in all cases the cats have shared the same good health as their canine counterparts.

It is over fifty years since I pioneered seaweed as an important food supplement for animals of all kinds, cats included. In recent years, seaweed has been universally accepted as useful and important for all domestic creatures, including poultry for which it is particularly good as an egg-laying tonic, and one can now buy dozens of brands. More recently, I have been pioneering other modern food supplements: bran, of course (but natural bran, not the 'fancy' breakfast cereal form), also carob pods and coconut, both in powder form.

To benefit from such foods a cat would require a small teaspoon of each, added to other food, most days of the week. Both dogs and cats enjoy carob and coconut, but seaweed taste is not palatable to them and should be disguised in other food.

Before I give the Natural Rearing diet for cats and kittens, it is necessary for me to pass on some carefully collected cat lore so that the domestic feline of both sexes may be better understood and appreciated.

In addition, I want to advise, if only briefly, on the general care of cats.

The American cat lover and expert, author Jean Harper, writes some very quotable words on cats in her interesting book, *The Healthy Cat and Dog Cook Book* (Soodik, USA):

Cats have been companions to mankind for thousands of years. In Egypt they were sacred symbols. In Siam they guarded the royal palace . . . No picture of the family hearth is really right without the family cat curled up and exuding a feeling of warmth and comfort. Cats are easy to care for; they are by nature strong and very self-reliant.

I really must emphasize that cat strength comes from Nature

because cats, since they were first domesticated, have enjoyed far greater freedom than dogs. And they need this continuing freedom if they are to retain their typical strength. They need to exercise themselves fully in meadow prowling and tree climbing if country cats, and roof-top and alley prowling if city cats. The neutered cats confined to city apartments are usually sorry specimens of the true feline. How can such cats obtain the natural fresh grasses, roots and tree barks needed to keep them healthy, or catch the wild prey which is their most natural food and which they are so skilled in catching, whether it be large insects or rodents? How can they fulfil themselves if they are permanent prisoners indoors? Indoors, the most they would catch would be an occasional moth or mouse!

The cat, because of its tiger lineage, being a descendant of the great cats, is a wholehearted sun lover and to be deprived of sunlight, kept closed away in some dark apartment into which the sun never enters, is true punishment for any cat.

If city cats have to be confined (they never used to be; the acrobatic cat was once a feature of city life as it chased around), then they can be taught to take exercise, dog-like, on collar and leash. But it is necessary to start their leash training early, from kittenhood.

I well recall meeting a Spanish gypsy woman in a woodland beyond Malaga in Andalucia. She was of the true nomad type, a real foot traveller. On her endless travels she took along with her, not her human family but an animal family – two cats and two dogs. The cats walked by her side controlled by leashes and collars (they all wore jingling bells) and when they became tired their owner lifted them up into a basket which she carried hooked over her left arm and into which the cats settled contentedly.

In Greece I have seen many true wild cats of the lonely places, savage, cruel-clawed creatures, able to rear their litters of kittens in wonderful health, subsisting entirely on foods self-taken from the sea-coast pools and from the inland fields and woodlands.

The most impressive wild cats I have ever seen were in Holland, in the moorlands of Drenthe. Heavy snow brought them to our farm to steal grain from the bins and hunt the granary mice. Because those cats were heavily long-haired, I expect they were domestic animals who had taken to the woods, preferring the life of the wild.

What beautiful fiery-eyed creatures they were and with what suppleness and rhythm they moved: so wild! They were impossible to photograph, though I had tried to do so, for the merest sound of a human foot on the snow and they sped away out of sight. They remained around the farm for many weeks and littered the snow with fur and feathers from the prey they had caught when humans were out of the way.

The common ailments of the domestic cat of earlier times were as few and simple as those of the dog, but nowadays, due to man's mismanagement of cat care, the provision of easily prepared canned and packet foods, curtailed exercise and the air and water pollution all around us, the cat, like the dog, suffers from a huge list of painful ailments, many of which are quick killers. Just take a few of the modern ones, all of which are prevalent: feline panleukopenia (feline distemper), hepatitis, feline infectious peritonitis, salmonella, feline leukaemia, etc.

All these ailments can be effectively treated in cats as in dogs, using herbal natural cures which concentrate on fasting, the use of hydromel (honey and water) and of the appropriate herbs for individual complaints. As I have already pointed out, the canine veterinary treatments will also help the cat, but use smaller dosages.

One stands a far better chance of a cure by using simple herbal remedies than by treatments with unnatural chemicals. The chemicals mostly aim at just reducing the symptoms by suppressive measures, despite the fact that a high temperature is very often created specially by the body in order to burn up the invading bacteria. Thus, sudden reduction of fever by chemicals defeats the self-healing processes of the body and can do serious harm. I have written about all this in my veterinary canine writings and all of it applies equally to the cat.

Some final remarks are helpful to the cat. Do let every house cat have its own special 'den', a place in the quietest part of the house where it can go and rest when inclined, and go to sleep when sleep is wanted. I stress 'quiet' because the ears of the cat are supersensitive (almost owl- and falcon-like in this respect) and the general noise of the modern home, with radio, video and television all in use, will be a true affliction for the cat's hearing. Provide a box or basket, line it with some comfortable cotton padding (not nylon or wool) and put this in a quiet dimly lit place for the cat to have its 'tiger den'. I prefer a box to a basket because, although a basket is much more attractive to have in one's home, baskets do harbour that persistent and parasitical insect, the cat flea. The small, black, cat flea is much more difficult to control than the larger, brown, dog flea, and the cat flea is more prone to bite humans, and very difficult to eradicate once it has invaded human dwellings: therefore take care to keep fleas under control.

If the domestic cat is allowed to wander about at will, it will obtain most of its needs in medicinal herbs. The cat is not quite the super-skilled self-herbalist that the dog is, but is quite efficient none the less.

Remember the cat's special love of the herb *Nepeta* of the Labiatae, or mint, family. The cat chews at this plant and also likes to roll itself on it. The cat makes a good choice in its favourite as *Nepeta cataria* (catmint or catnip) is very medicinal, being a powerful herb tonic and one of the best-known remedies against diabetes, both prevention and cure.

The cat's 'rollin' in the mint' frolic is not just for pleasure; it is also the feline cunning for disguise. The strong odour of *Nepeta* disguises the cat's own body smell so that prey which it is seeking to kill and eat will not be aware, by scent on the wind, of the cat stalking it.

Like the big cats – tigers and leopards – the domestic cat is also a dedicated sunbather, so for health's sake do see that your cat has access to all the sunlight it desires.

A book by Roger Tabor called *The Wild Life of the Domestic Cat* (Arrow Books, England) tells how the home cat has persisted in retaining many of its former wild-life habitats. The book was reviewed in the BBC 'Nature Notebook' weekly programme and made a great impression on me. It aroused my sympathy for this independent creature, the cat, when it is held captive by modern man.

All who own and love cats should make sure that their pets can retain some of this 'wildness' by allowing them the freedoms: freedom to prowl and hunt to catch some food for themselves; freedom to mate and raise a family; freedom to know the night which is the cat's true time – it is a nocturnal creature by character and skills. All these are sorely needed for real mental and bodily health.

NATURAL REARING DIET FOR CATS

The five main rules of Natural Rearing are:

1 Correct natural diet of mainly raw foods.
2 Abundant fresh air and sunlight.
3 Much active outdoor exercise.
4 Avoidance of 'animal-sick' (over-used) land.

5 Provision of couch grass and catmint (*Nepeta cataria*) as basic cat medicine.

KITTENS

It is impossible to advise exact amounts of food to be given because this is influenced by several factors. Exercise, temperament, breed of cat, climate, all affect the appetite of adult cats as well as kittens. If the animal's stomach distends after meals, then smaller meals should be given. Kittens should have individual dishes and should remain on milk foods only until near four weeks old, but they can be offered other milk, fortified with honey, to help their mothers' milk. From two weeks of age they should have access to fresh drinking water.

Weaning

From four weeks of age: Supplement mother's milk with:

8 a.m.: Milk, preferably raw, fresh milk, not dried or long-life milks and preferably not pasteurized. Fortify with NR gruel (tree barks and plant roots), a small teaspoon per kitten. Kittens weaned on to this will, as adults, also enjoy milk and gruel; otherwise some cats will not take milk after weaning and milk is a most useful cat food.
12 noon: Repeat the 8 a.m. meal without the gruel. Add a teaspoon of flaked cereals.
4 p.m.: Repeat 12 noon meal.
8 p.m.: Repeat 8 a.m. meal.

After six weeks of age: Confine milk meals to morning: 8 a.m. and noon. Feed several teaspoons of raw meat or lightly baked fish (both meat and fish scraped with sharp knife or finely cut, not minced) at 4 and 8 p.m. Add a pinch of NR seaweed, etc, blend powder and a teaspoon of finely minced raw salad greens such as parsley, mint, celery, cresses, dandelion (several preferably).

Note: Kittens (unlike puppies) may require more frequent meals in their early weeks of weaning.

After weaning to four months of age

8 a.m.: As much of the usual 8 a.m. meal (milk with gruel) as the kittens will eat. Now include a sprinkle of flaked cereals.

12 noon: Omit gruel from milk and thicken with such health cereals as blended flakes and some NR (Puppy and Junior) Meal, which contains such health fortifiers as powdered malt, liquorice, carob, etc, or obtain your own and add.

Add also a few drops of vegetable oil, preferably sunflower, corn (maize) or sesame. Beaten raw egg can be given on some days. Cottage cheese is another healthful food that is good for cats. A small sprinkle of desiccated (powdered) coconut can be given because it contains the rare ingredient albumin, is mineral rich and deters worms.

4 p.m.: Meat: a few dessertspoons or more depending on appetite, shredded into small pieces, never minced. Breast of mutton can be given including the bones: meat without bones is unnatural. Give only a small amount of fat; always remember that the body, in self-defence, isolates pesticides, pollutants and other foreign matter in body fat. Add a teaspoon of pure bran, raw for extra fibre because butcher's meat is supplied without skin with hair, and a pinch of minerals blend of seaweed and land plants. A teaspoon of mixed salad greens – garden and wild and the bigger the variety the better – can be added, but they must be very finely cut because felines have difficulty in digesting cellulose. *The inclusion of raw greens in diet is vital to health.* Further useful additions are minced sprouted grains and pulses, finely grated carrot and grated raw apple, given several days in the week.

FISH   Can quite frequently replace part of the meat suggested in the NR diet. Cats have a keen liking for fish and on my travels I have often seen them – particularly the wild ones – scooping fish out of streams and pools and eating them raw. Fresh-caught fish can be fed to domestic cats raw. Otherwise plunge it into boiling water, steam it lightly, or bake it. Do not fry fish and do not use canned fish.

POULTRY and RABBIT   These also can take the place of meat. If freshly killed they can be given raw, otherwise plunge them into boiling water or they can be lightly baked. But remember that *raw is best*.

CANNED FOODS   These should be avoided at all costs, particularly canned meats and canned fish. All canned foods are without any guarantee of origin, some come from unclean sources, and most of them contain chemical preservatives. Do remember that Natural Rearing means natural foods – avoid the unnatural.

Note: Cats should have flesh foods on only four or five days of the week because no wild animal could possibly kill prey daily! In the wild there must be days of little food. Therefore feed domestic animals very sparsely for two days in every week, few meals and lighter ones, semi-fasting should be the idea. On those days feed only milky cereals, minced greens, diluted cottage cheese.

At four months of age: Fewer meals can be given if preferred, leaving out the midday meal.

At eight months, or a little later: The adult cat diet can be followed.

Note: Every kitten from weaning onward should rest and cleanse its internal organs frequently by fasts on plain water only. No kitten should be tempted or coaxed to eat and food not eaten promptly should be removed. Every kitten over three months old should have a half-day fast once a week, Sunday for instance, and a whole-day fast once a month.

Do not prevent kittens from eating clean earth and sand and small stones; they often eat such things instinctively for minerals and trace elements and to remove worms. The same advice applies to the excreta of grassfed animals – sheep, goats, cattle, etc. This is quite natural for carnivores.

Cats should also be encouraged to eat charcoal and any green herb, particularly couch grass (also known as twitch, crab grass, dog grass), that common weed and a basic internal cleanser for the carnivores, used as a laxative or to induce cleansing vomiting. Cats will also eat other medicinal herbs such as mosses, lichens, rough leaves of comfrey and borage, leaves of oats and maize and so on. They also show a great liking for cucumbers and melons, the seeds of which are a further internal cleanser and tonic, and enjoy sweet corn finely grated, raw, or lightly cooked (only the young, fresh cobs are suitable when the kernels are very milky): this is an excellent tonic and promotes good hair.

Never feed to any animal hot food or very cold (refrigerated) food: both are unnatural and can provoke cancer of the tongue, throat, etc, right down to the anus.

A VARIED DIET FOR HEALTH It is as well to remember that cats get a variety of foods from the intestines and stomach contents of their prey. Cats in the wild prey on herbivore creatures such as birds and rodents and from their inner organs obtain healthful vegetable matter – grains, fruits and nuts (in crushed form).

Give sometimes brown rice with lentils, for iron and vitamins. Give also a sprinkle of bran for extra roughage. Try and buy organic bran because the outside of cereals are generally sprayed with pesticides.

BONES   All cats love meaty bones, but are often deprived of them by their owners because of fears that they might cause choking or internal damage. Bones are vital for health of teeth and jaws and for the entire internal system, as well as for pleasure in their eating and playing with them. But do not misuse bones: never cook them as this renders them apt to split into sharp pieces and points. Also, do not give bones on an empty stomach, give them at the end of a meal. Avoid hide (buffalo, etc) bones and plastic bones from pet shops – dangerous.

VINEGAR   When cats seem to be stiff limbed and 'arthriticky', add a teaspoon of apple or wine vinegar (no other) to their drinking water for five days in a week.

WATER   Provide fresh drinking water day and night and not in a plastic dish.

DIET FOR ADULT CATS

Most cats enjoy a light breakfast of bread and whole-grain cereals in milk, wholewheat bread lightly buttered or spread with white cheese cut small.

Otherwise follow the same diet as for kittens with the midday and 8 p.m. meals given later in each case.

This may sound a complicated way of feeding kittens and

cats compared with the common, seemingly orthodox, diet of a can of fish or meat of popular make and well commercialized, and a packet of processed cereals made totally lifeless.

But Natural Rearing diet has long been proved as far cheaper because animals raised in this way need far less food and have the strength and vitality to catch much of their own food from the fields (wild rabbits in particular) if allowed the freedom to do so.

Surely it makes sense to feed a diet natural to the kitten and cat, based on their former wild life, rather than to have to pay out large sums of money in an attempt to cure cats of the ever-growing number of true horror ailments which now 'belong' to the domestic cat of our unnatural modern times and which kill off thousands of domestic animals annually.

For proof of this statement, look at any modern cat-care book and read the long list of ailments with strange-sounding names which afflict animals fed on 'quick and easy' meals instead of on slower, more time-taking, healthier ones.

RODENTS The cat, being a night animal, is able to see perfectly in the dark and so is a principal killer and eater of rodents. In fact, many people and farmers in particular keep cats to rid themselves of destructive rodents. Unfortunately this brings cats into the danger zone of eating poison indirectly through the bodies of their prey. Some cats will merely kill rodents, not eat them.

The other skilled killers of rodents are birds of prey, mostly owls of all kinds and many species of hawk. It is a sad fact that each year hundreds of cats and birds die as a result of poisoning.

The best and most sensible way to control rodents is prevent their access to foods which they like and to water wherever possible. Otherwise, catch them in traps or hunt them down with rat-catcher type dogs such as the smaller terrier breeds, although it is of interest to note that Afghan hounds are expert catchers of rats and mice. Poison, besides being extremely painful to the consumer, is not successful in controlling rodents as the huge and ever-growing world population of vermin confirms. It fails because the rat is a creature of infinite cunning and is selective. The less intelligent rats eat poison and die, but the cleverest avoid it and survive to breed ever more cunning rats. Treatment for poisoning, including rat poison, is given elsewhere in this book.

OILS The oils advised for use in cat food – sesame, corn or sunflower – are important to diet because they supply vitamins and minerals.

Finally, and the most important piece of all advice about felines:

CAT CLAWS (taken from my new book, *Cats – Naturally: Natural Rearing for Healthier Cats*) Its claws are *vital* to the cat. Despite its small size and weight, the cat is a valiant fighter. Without its claws a cat becomes a defenceless creature.

Formerly, it was not necessary to advise on cat claws, other than keeping them in good condition by oiling and trimming. Now there is a new and terrible development concerning cat claws. Modern cat owners in ever-increasing numbers are having a cruel, painful, and often dangerous operation performed on their cats, the operation known as *de-clawing*.

This is done to prevent cats from scratching their owners and for protection of household furnishings and wood!

This veterinary operation of de-clawing is the equivalent of cutting off the last joint of every finger of the human hand, to which cat claws are similar.

Cats use their claws not only for killing prey for their food, but for other purposes such as the exercise of leg muscles brought into use when cats are stretching and contracting and pressing with their claws. These are needed for daily grooming, which is an important part of feline life. With their claws they open up hair mats, remove skin parasites, and pull away irritant and often painful and harmful vegetation which has become attached to their hair.

They also make use of their claws when eating food, tearing up portions of flesh, rendering it small enough to enter their mouths, and for lifting food into their mouths and holding it there to chew, cats having only small mouths and not very powerful teeth.

Fortunately, indeed very fortunately, the de-clawing operation is costly and difficult to perform. Furthermore, it is painful to the animal and many veterinarians advise against it and refuse to do it. The high cost does deter the general cat-owner, but many owners who choose to have their cats de-clawed do not realize the harm they are doing. It is the duty of every veterinarian to inform cat-owners fully.

The de-clawed cat, aware of its defenceless state and greatly handicapped, may become permanently mentally depressed and unbalanced and will never again be the happy, purring, domestic cat.

Indoors, cats should be given special scratching places and be taught to use them. Such scratching posts can be purchased from well-equipped pet shops.

As for cats scratching their owners, my advice is never to try and hold a cat by force against its will, when it wants to get away from human hands. Let the cat go, rather than turn it into a scratcher, and do not try to take food away from a cat when it is eating: it may scratch to protect its food.

5

General Notes on Natural Rearing

Throughout the preceding chapters of this book I have stressed the importance of diet in puppy rearing, for without proper diet you cannot rear healthy puppies. It is nonsense, for example, to advise adequate exercise if the puppy's limbs have been rendered too rachitic (rickety) from faulty diet to allow any exercise to be taken.

But in this chapter, assuming that proper diet is being followed, I am giving some well-proved hints on puppy care which will add to the well-being of all puppies. I have followed the plan of a book on horse breeding which I once used to study; this book was divided into two sections: 'The External Horse' and 'The Internal Horse'.

The external dealt with grooming, stable management, exercise, and so forth; the internal with diet, disease prevention and cure. I shall in this chapter follow something of that horse-book plan.

ALL THE ADVICE GIVEN IS SUITABLE FOR CATS.

EXTERNAL CARE

GROOMING   Daily grooming is an essential of puppy rearing when stock is kennel raised. Yet I have known famous kennels (famous on show wins only) who never groom their stock except for show preparation. Grooming encourages hair growth, allows the hair – which, after all, is a living tissue – to breathe, keeps vermin in check, aids the circulation, and conditions the delicate nerve fibres which mass in the skin layers. Country-living dogs require less grooming than town ones, for in their daily exercise the herbage and bushes friction their bodies, and clean rain bathes them. They are also able to roll themselves on grass. Only in summertime they must be searched for skin vermin, especially grass ticks. I advocate for all dogs a weekly sponge-down with pine fluid (genuine, not synthetic), a few drops to a half pint of tepid water, and a monthly bath in soapy water, rinsing off very well. Use soap flakes, not detergents, and a bar of olive oil soap, such as Palmolive. More frequent bathing is essential for town dogs, grimed by chimney smoke and motor-vehicle fumes. No dog can enjoy true health when its body is coated with a film of grime.

An Afghan hound I had with me for three months in New York required a weekly bath; and each week tubs of black, grimy water were washed from her golden coat.

Needless to say, all grooming equipment must also be washed at least weekly. It is useless to groom an animal with soiled combs and brushes. Bristle brushes and bone combs are far better for hair health than plastic ones. Collars and leads should also be cleaned regularly, using an oily or paraffin rag, and then polishing with a good leather polish.

Dogs must be examined regularly for presence of lice, fleas, ticks, or mange infections. Coats should be dusted frequently with a safe herbal insecticide. Never use poisons. They not only harm the eyes and inner ears of dogs, but also settle on herbage and contaminate food, and act as insidious, if slow, poisons internally. For fuller instructions for safe destruction of skin vermin, see 'Fleas, Lice, Ticks, etc', in Chapter 7. For years I used a non-toxic bathing block, called Canex, made in Israel; a total killer of fleas. But the weight of the block made it non-commercial for selling by post and it is no longer available.

Using the same principle of foamy suffocation of fleas and a herbal oil to compel them to the hair surface, I have evolved a successful flea-killer which is harmless in use to all types of animal. Make a bathing lotion as follows: take a cupful of *non-poisonous* washing-up liquid, choosing one which claims to be 'kind to the hands'. (I have found Palmolive to be reliable.) To every cup of detergent add two teaspoons of oil of eucalyptus and mix well.

Now wet the dog thoroughly, soaking the hair well. Next rub some of the lotion deeply into the hair to reach the skin. See that all parts of the animal are treated thoroughly, especially the ears, but keep out of the eyes. If it does enter, soothe at once by pouring in some fresh (not Long-life type) milk. Rinse off the lather thoroughly and apply a second time. Allow the lather to remain five minutes, rubbing in well all the time. Finally, rinse off very well and partly dry the animal with towels. Then stand it on a sheet of white paper and brush its hair thoroughly to bring out the dead fleas. Search the hair for any fleas which may have escaped the lather; they will be in a feeble state and can be killed with ease. I regret the use of a detergent, but its bitter-tasting foam is needed for such a foe as the flea!

Clean rain-water is a wonderful hair tonic, as also is dew. Exercise dogs in the rain frequently: a healthy dog loves rain. Dry down wet dogs with a dry wash-leather, which will absorb much moisture; newspaper can then be used to finish off, or handfuls of pine sawdust on smooth-coated dogs. Then bed the dog on thick layers of newspaper which will dry him off completely. Wet cats should also be bedded on newspaper for drying them. A dog loves to cleanse itself as nature intended, by rolling its body on grass, but this cannot be achieved if the grass is that of a stale kennel run, urine soaked and dirty. My Afghan hounds, retaining their natural instincts from their mountain-living ancestors, take self-taught grooming sessions by rolling among thickets of fern or on clumps of reeds. They do this deliberately, generation after generation. They also bath, rolling and kicking, in dry sand, which helps remove skin parasites.

For grooming 'shine' on coats, an excellent daily finish-off to grooming is friction and polishing with a wash-leather dipped into cold common tea or a strong brew of rosemary herb; best for dark coats, could stain light ones. Or the bare hands can be dipped into tea or herbal brew and used to polish the coat; that is how the Arabs polish their Arabian horses and salukis, using often a weak brew of henna leaves. Nettle tea is also a famous old-fashioned coat tonic, used as a friction, making the hair shine and removing scurf. (Some nettle tea can also be given with benefit for internal use, by spoon or soaked into the cereal feed. Bring nettles to the near boil in hot water, then remove from the boil and steep for two to three hours. Gloves must be used when cutting off the nettles, for they sting the skin at a touch before being cooked.)

SUNLIGHT   As I have said elsewhere in this book, without sun there can be no life. The maximum of sun for all animals should be a kennel rule, with ample shade provided too, so that the dog can himself choose his own natural sunbathing hours or seek shade, as he desires. Sunlight is not merely a tonic and restorative and a potent destroyer of bacteria, it is also a vital food. It is one of the main sources of vitamins A and D. It is understood that when a dog is seen to lick at its body hair after sunning itself, it is partaking of vitamin A, which collects on the hair surfaces; the dog is also seeking vital cosmic dust which comes earthward on the sun's rays. *Sunlight is essential to natural puppy rearing*; there is no substitute for it, not electric sunlamps or anything else. Puppies reared indoors in apartments or sometimes even below ground level in basements, as often happens in big cities in America and elsewhere, can never possess true health, and their disease resistance is very low.

KENNELS For Nature Rearing, kennels must be roomy, well ventilated, sunny, and dry. Artificial heating should be avoided; dogs, being of the wolf family, thrive in cold, but dislike damp. In very hot weather, the best dry warmth that man can provide for the domestic dog is a deep bed of dry litter, straw, hay, bracken, etc, in a draught-proof corner of the kennel. Pinewood sawdust or shavings on the floor give warmth and absorb damp. Long-coated breeds cannot have such bedding because it tangles in their coats. Thick layers of newspaper can be used, topped off with sacks. Wash sacks frequently because they can harbour fleas and lice. Rain-proofed roofs of kennels can cause uncomfortable heat inside during the summer months if there are prolonged spells of hot weather. Dogs cannot express their distress but they hate hot kennels and really suffer. To avoid such discomfort, make a habit of putting sacks soaked in cold water over kennel roofs when the sun is beating down, or they should be hosed with cold water several times a day. Concrete runs also get painfully hot and need to be cooled down. I never use concrete in any place that I keep my dogs or goats.

Winter litters are unnatural. The female fox and wolf will not mate in the mid-year; they await the natural breeding time which ensures springtime whelping, to rear their whelps in the warmth of spring sunlight. If some heat is needed for young puppies which have been winter whelped, then a paraffin-burning storm lantern, hung on a strong, long nail, to keep the lamp out of near contact with the wall, can be kept burning night and day. Make sure it is *very* secure because of fire danger. A storm lamp will give ample heat for any average size kennel. Keep the lamp spotlessly clean, allowing no drop of paraffin to remain on it after filling, to cause fume smells. In the coldest mountain winters of Spain I have never needed any other heating for my animals. When electricity is available, use a kennel lamp-heater hanging in an entirely safe position.

KENNEL RUNS Daily contact for long periods with clean earth and grassland is another essential of puppy NR. I have known puppies, fed strictly on raw foods and conditioned only with herbal medicines, who still did not thrive, solely because they were being kept in stale kennel runs soiled and worm infested by countless earlier litters. Puppies need a fresh or well-rested area of ground for each litter bred. Portable wire runs on wooden posts should be used with the wire moved to a different piece of land every month while the puppies are young and constantly soiling the runs. Paint all wood frequently with creosote. Unlike that of cattle, sheep and goats, the urine of dogs is bad for the soil. Stale earth runs should be dug over and well limed and then sown with fresh lawn-making grass seed. I have known grass seed to refuse to grow at all in much-used dog runs, even after liming, so foul and sour had the earth been allowed to become. No wonder, therefore, that puppies reared in such runs grow up to be sickly creatures, undersized and nervous. Plant clumps of couch grass in the runs, as canine medicine. Encourage earthworms in the runs, as their presence in the ground helps to decompose the dangerous eggs of worms, tapeworm segments and flea eggs. The nature farmers' policy of cropping paddocks heavily with mustard and then ploughing it into the ground as an earth disinfectant is also an excellent policy for the cleansing of kennel runs.

Miss A.N. Hartley, Rotherwood Deerhounds, who has

reared so many stalwart champion hounds in this country, sums up the matter very well in a letter to me:

> Cleanliness, fresh air and exercise, and good food, have always been my four essentials of puppy rearing. I agree with you most heartily in believing that having too many dogs on a small area spells inevitable disaster. The dogs and runs are consequently not then kept really clean, with the result that bacteria find good living quarters.
>
> Far too many people believe that dog breeding is a pleasant hobby with which to make money in one's spare time, and this spells overcrowding and neglect of the dogs.

Vernon Hirst, famed English terrier man and judge, gives sound advice:

> I am a believer in letting my bitches and puppies run on natural ground, and did not have my runs concreted. I used to place a nice-sized board inside the run for them to lie on when at rest in good weather. I used to keep as near to the natural as possible, and the result was I escaped many illnesses.

CHAINING   Above all else, never leave a dog chained. I have seen the chained ones everywhere on my travels: in English town yards and on farms, on Spanish and Mexican farms, as protectors of factories and lonely properties in America, and guarding barracks and arms dumps in Israel. In most cases they were described as 'watchdogs'. One day all chaining will be made illegal; certainly it is unnatural

Some years ago on a Greek island I saw a small brown pointer bitch tied to a tree during an entire month. She was still tied there when I left Greece. The tree did not give much shade, therefore by day sunlight burned her and by night the cold of that region froze her. Her food was true prison fare:

stale bread and water only. She lay in her own excreta, tormented by flies, visited by rats wanting the stale bread. Her despairing howls disturbed the neighbouring farms, but no one interfered. If I had freed her, doglike she would have run back miles to where her owner lived, only to be beaten and returned to the tree. If I'd stolen her to get her to kinder hands, she would have been found by the police when I tried to leave the island with her. Dreadful cruelty!

EXERCISE Early-morning and evening exercise is best. Do not exercise in the full heat of a summer day or immediately after meals. For true health, allow all dogs to enjoy exercise in all weathers, wind, rain, snow. Leash exercise is almost valueless. A dog needs to run and leap, and thus fill its lungs with an abundance of oxygen. Unfortunately, many dogs have to breathe the stale air of cities. Dogs will not exercise themselves fully in paddocks or runs, they will be apt to sit around waiting for the greater freedom offered by natural exercise outside their confines. Abundant daily exercise is needed for full digestion of a carnivorous diet. Also blood circulation is never normal in any dog denied its natural running freedom. Likewise, the organs of the body concerned with circulation – the lungs, heart, arteries, and veins – will diminish in strength with every passing year, until there will come the time when dogs will become semi-invalid years before their time, and no longer able to run tirelessly as the natural fox or wolf runs. The nervous system also becomes disordered, rendering the dog snappy or over-excited, or yapping or barking incessantly and without reason, typical of many kennel dogs. Also the coats of dogs lacking exercise are dull and often smell strongly because the blood which feeds the hair is sluggish.

If one lives near the sea let dogs enjoy healthful sea-bathing. Euripides, the Greek naturalist and teacher, taught wisely that 'The Sea cures all the ills of man.' It is likewise a real benefit for animals. Many racehorses are walked daily in shallow sea-water to strengthen their legs: I also walk my Afghan hounds when we live by the sea, which is our usual environment.

If the sea in which dogs bathe is the now generally polluted water, take the dog home and wash down by pouring over the dog several buckets of slightly warmed tap water to wash the coat free of any sea pollution. Dogs are natural swimmers and have been known to rescue drowning humans. The Newfoundland breed is particularly credited with this.

DISCIPLINE This is also of importance to total health. A wise observation: the bitch trains her whelps for nine weeks, then man takes over for around nineteen years. Human will-power concentrated on an animal's will, together with loving sympathy and strict daily routine, are the essentials for contented dogs. A young puppy should be trained from the time of weaning to the following requirements: (1) to respond to its own name; (2) to return when called; (3) to be clean in kennel habits; (4) not to steal or be greedy when feeding; (5) not to be quarrelsome with fellow dogs; (6) to be friendly towards people but not to fawn; (7) not to whine or bark without real reason; (8) to guard when needed.

To bring out friendliness in kennel puppies, take them in turn into the home for visits. I like the words in *The Animals Charter*, published by International Cultural Forum (UK branch, 127 Nevill Avenue, Hove, Sussex, England):

> May they [human beings] talk to us sometimes and give us their companionship realizing that in order to share their lives *we have for the most part to forgo the society of our own kind* – thus delivering us from the suffering due to loneliness and lack of fellowship.

A dog in its natural state would never soil its bed or yelp unceasingly without reason: it is man who has turned so many dogs into such unpleasant and dirty creatures.

Puppies should not be allowed to chew indiscriminately at anything they choose; they must be taught to exercise their teeth on suitable objects. The gypsies give roots for chewing to their greyhound or lurcher puppies, especially marshmallow roots, also cabbage stumps. I have found a twisted coil of rope gives good jaw exercise. Do not leave old bones lying around for mice and rats to contaminate or for flies to breed on.

Once the habit of house or kennel dirtying with urine or excreta has been acquired, the breaking of the habit is not easy. Put pepper on places where puppies have soiled; they will not return to the same place then. When puppies refuse to relieve themselves outdoors, to induce them to have a bowel action an infant-size suppository can be used several times, or the fleshy stalk of a plant can be inserted into the anus. When the puppy has had a bowel action, it can then be much patted in praise and taken at once back into the house. Use the same words each time when the puppy is required to have a bowel action. Soon the puppy understands what is required of him and there is no further trouble. This is the simplest way to house-train a puppy. Do not use the hand to strike in punishment. The hand should be a symbol of love, for the handing out of food and drink, for caresses, for attaching to the leash for the pleasure of exercise, and for freeing from the leash for the greater joy of unhampered running. When punishment is truly needed – and this should be very rare – then use a folded magazine or a supple slipper. Strike an animal on the legs, never on the head or back.

INTERNAL CARE

This subject is mostly dealt with in the chapters on weaning, puppy diet, etc. However, it is my intention to include a few odd notes on puppy ailments and allied subjects not previously dealt with.

COUGHING This is a common symptom of distemper, or worms, or both. In olden times, distemper was described as 'the husk'. Immediate treatment consists of: fasting on honey-water, dosing with garlic or herbal tablets, or a strong brew of onions if the garlic is not available for immediate use. Elder blossom or berries, or sage, in a brew are also good. Temperature should be taken. Treatment details are given under Coughing, pages 167-8.

DEPRAVED APPETITE This malady refers to the unhealthy habit of a puppy eating its own or other puppies' excreta. The eating of herbivorous droppings, cow pats, rabbit pellets, etc, is quite normal and healthful, and is only a typical canine search for extra herbal and mineral matter. But carnivorous excreta is highly toxic and harmful, and such a depraved eating habit must be checked. Worm infestation is a common cause, also boredom – especially lack of exercise. Canine faeces, in any case, should not be left lying on the ground to breed flies or spread parasitical worm ova; they should be removed promptly many times daily. When exercising my hounds on leash, I always cover their excreta with earth or stones to prevent flies. Of course this cannot be done on town pavements, but at least dogs can be led into the street off the pavement when excreting. Treatment of faeces-eating consists of putting paraffin on the excreta to cause a repellent taste. There is also internal treatment, by increasing mineral

120

intake with the feeding of twice the usual amount of daily seaweed powder given with the meat feed until the cure is complete; supplying daily a large raw bone to chew at; adding black treacle or molasses to the milk feed. It is also depraved appetite when a dog refuses raw meat and wants only cooked or canned food. Fast until *natural* food is accepted.

DIARRHOEA   (See pp. 83–4, 169–71.)

DISCHARGING EYES This may be a symptom of worms or distemper. Temperature of the puppy should be taken. The eyes should be bathed with a brew of common chamomile or fennel or balm leaves. A mixture of milk with the herbal brew is very effective; also witch hazel: one part herbal brew, a half teaspoon each of witch hazel and milk to every two table-spoons of herb. The brews of elder blossom or chickweed or ground ivy are good, soothing eye treatments, also the juice of raw cucumbers, squeezed into the eyes to remedy inflammation.

DISTEMPER   (See Chapter 7.)

EATING FOREIGN BODIES Puppies will eat wire, glass, tin, rubber, and other remarkable things often out of sheer playful-ness. The best remedy is a meal of bread and milk, to mix around the foreign body, followed by a stiff dose of castor oil. For splinters of cooked bones – highly dangerous – lumps of cotton wool, not big enough to risk choking, can be rammed down the throat to wrap around the object; a laxative dose of castor oil should follow later. (See also Poison, for method of inducing immediate vomiting.)

FITS, HYSTERIA (See Chapter 7.) Immediate treatment is isolation in a quite place. Stoppage of all food, fasting on honey-water diet. A daily laxative.

NAVEL HERNIA When bitches have a nervous whelping, they may drag around one or two of the first-born pups, leaving behind a lump where the navel cord was attached. As soon as the cord stump has withered the lump should be pressed back into the inner body, using pressure of the thumb. This usually gives an instant cure, but, if necessary, massage with a strong brew of ivy leaves fortified with astringent witch hazel.

POISON (See Chapter 7.) Puppies will eat such things as matches, poisoned vermin, and so on. A piece of washing soda about the size of a small bean pushed down the throat will cause immediate vomiting. Larger breeds require several pieces of soda to produce vomiting. (*Make sure* dangerous caustic soda is not given in mistake for washing soda.) Another emetic is vinegar and mustard: approximately two teaspoons of vinegar to every teaspoon of mustard, spooned down the throat – an approximate quarter to half cupful of the mixture for an average size dog. A stiff emetic may also be made from table salt in water, several teaspoons of salt. Give castor oil, a strong dose, as an immediate laxative.

RICKETS This ailment is 100 per cent preventable, and is mostly due to unnatural rearing conditions. The predominant fault is unhealthy diet, especially the feeding of cooked and denatured foods. Additional faults are overcrowded kennel accommodation, lack of sunlight, and lack of contact with clean grassland; over-early weaning is also a cause.

Of what use is a dog without strong legs? And yet so many modern dogs possess malformed legs or shelly boned ones.

On sound puppy rearing – which means strong-boned stock – rests the whole future of a breed of dog. The health record of many of the best-known English and American breeds, at the present time, is not an enviable one; most breeds have quite a formidable list of hereditary ailments, specific ailments typifying the different breeds, the worst health records being among the oldest-established European breeds.

The one sure prescription for cure of rickets and general health improvement is to adopt fully Natural Rearing. The best herbal remedies for cure of rickets are: raw carrot, parsley, comfrey, and seaweed. Slippery-elm bark also should be used, as in the Natural Rearing gruel.

SICKNESS Vomiting in the dog should always be encouraged; it is Nature's way of causing prompt internal cleansing. Vomiting following the eating of couch grass, mustard leaves, lichens, etc, is deliberate and cleansing.

SORE FOOT PADS (See Sore Pads, Chapter 7.)

STINGS These are really external, but can be dealt with here. They are not dangerous except when on the tongue. Many puppies have a habit of snapping at wasps and bees. After removing the sting, the area should be rubbed immediately with a piece of washing soda, dipped in water. This alkaline substance neutralizes the acid of the sting. A slice of raw onion or garlic can also be used, or vinegar or raw lemon juice or witch hazel – any of these applied to the sting area. Ammonia or whitewash (lime) are further safe aids, diluted with three parts of water: for external use only, keep away from the eyes.

STOMACH SWELLING Frequent swelling of the stomach following meals often indicates worms, for which treatment see Worms, Chapter 7. However, overfeeding may also be the root cause. Stonehenge rightly says that 'art founded on experience' is required to fix the amount of food to give a growing puppy. The main test should be the eating up of all food greedily, no scouring, and no bloating. Puppies should still be active after each meal taken.

TEETHING   The first puppy teeth are milk teeth, appearing at four to five weeks of age, when the puppy is ready for solid foods. It should be a rule that no solids should be fed until the milk teeth first appear. These teeth eventually number twenty in the upper jaw, and twenty-two in the lower. They remain until the puppy is five to six months of age. No Natural Reared puppy ever develops teething fits or other teething ailments. Sound and easily produced teeth are a natural heritage of healthy puppies. But for those breeders who are new to NR, and have yet to produce NR stock, it should be emphasized that, should teething fits or other unnatural teething troubles occur, these should never be suppressed with chemicals. The puppy should be fasted for a day or two; dosed with a brew of skullcap or rosemary or sage, and the gums bathed twice daily with a brew of rosemary, or give poppy flower buds as pills, four buds twice daily, or a brew of field poppy flowers or poppy seed capsules, with honey.

WORMS   (See Chapters 3 and 7.)

And now this puppy-rearing part is almost at an end, and it will be noted that, except for a few minor infant ailments, dealt with in an earlier chapter, the ailments are few – and yet most books on animal rearing devote three-quarters of the work to dealing with disease treatment. I have not just forgotten about disease! However, *if dog owners will truthfully and strictly follow the rulings and the teachings of this book they will achieve what I have achieved with my Afghan hounds in England and elsewhere, and Sir Albert Howard with his cattle in India, and*

what numerous other breeders have achieved worldwide among their
dogs: disease-free and disease-immune stock.

But perfection is not built overnight. It took me many
generations of careful rearing before I could get my Afghans
up to a really high standard of health. Therefore, those
breeders who do meet with disease must follow the curative
treatments as given in Part Two of this book, in which all of
the common canine ailments – both puppy and adult – are
given in detail.

Breeders who experience sickness among their NR litters
should not become discouraged. Nature is a slow worker:
breeders are not going to get perfect, level, and unbroken
health before a fifth generation of NR. And when breeders
have to use outside stud dogs they are undoing much of the
good work (especially if such dogs are from inoculated stock).
Quite positively, among my Afghan hound litters after the
second generation I never had serious illness. But the Afghan
is a very 'natural' breed, which has not been spoiled by
Western rearing methods, at least not in the time that I was
raising my Turkuman litters. But, even so, occasional bouts of
bowel looseness, disinclination for food, and so on, are quite
a normal course of affairs in all infant rearing (children
included). There must be an ebb and flow of health; toxins
must accumulate from the very air (impure) that we breathe,
especially in or near cities, alone, and from milk and other
imperfect foods, even from cultivated vegetables which,
unlike most wild ones, are often far from perfect and know
disease themselves often enough; also think of today's prevalent low health standard of the animals upon whose flesh the
domesticated dog must be fed. A short period of fasting and
internal cleansing – usually a three-days' treatment – should
soon normalize things, and will give improved health. When,
of course, there is a deep infection, such as distemper, then
treatment must be more prolonged; but, correctly treated by

herbal methods, the disease will efficiently cleanse the organism and can only leave improved health. Disease awakens the latent healing powers of the body, tests them, and thereby strengthens them often enough. In rare cases disease treatment, by herbal medicine, may be prolonged into many months; many relapses may occur during treatment, but the final results will be total and permanent cure. Nature does not fail those who employ her diligently and faithfully.

Breeders having reared healthy puppies should then follow the principle of Mrs F.E. Nuhn, Manakiki Kennels, of German shepherds, Willoughby, Ohio, USA. 'My adults and puppies are maintained in such marvellous hard condition on Natural Rearing, following strictly as described in your books, that I am trying to educate my clientele to do as I do here or else they do not get a puppy!'

And when adding to their kennels, they should seek out NR stock in the manner of this Swiss doctor:

Dr Alexander Schleidt, of Halisberg, Bernese Oberland, wrote to me:

I am a faithful Swiss follower of your advice in your herbal books, which with your NR system has made my black and tan long-haired dachshunds so healthy, so full of pep, that they have become the terror of all neighbour dogs, foxes, badgers, hares, chamois, and deer, in the vicinity of our chalet! I now require a Pyrenean mountain dog as an extra guard, and since by long experience we know what wonderful results are obtained provided dogs are bred and kept according to your advice, I write to know of a kennel which follows the Natural Methods.

This letter came to me in April 1990 from Mr Geoffrey Fielding of Selston, Notts, England:

My mother had a collie cross bitch who, although being only three years old was diagnosed by vets as having an incurable cancer in the lower part of the throat, and they said the bitch should be put to sleep. However, after several weeks' treatment using violet leaves made into an infusion as directed in *The Complete Herbal Handbook for the Dog and Cat* [p. 136] she made a full recovery, gaining weight again and not vomiting, as had been the case. The tumour has now gone and the bitch is 100 per cent fit and well again, thanks to Juliette de Baîracli Levy's book. I write this letter with many thanks on behalf of my mother.

As for myself, I have trained racing greyhounds for twenty years and have had *great* success using both a natural diet and treatments from this book. Many thanks once again.

Now and then I get negative reports from readers. They state that despite following the method given in this book, results have been bad. When I was first teaching Natural Rearing (and herbal veterinary medicine) to the canine world, I used to visit dissatisfied readers to find out what had gone wrong. Invariably I found they were not following my book at all, or very incompletely! They were failing in diet (usually giving cooked meat and a large proportion of canned foods), thus breaking the basic rule of Natural Rearing – the raw foods diet. The vital, daily, inclusion of chopped raw greens was omitted. Or there was almost no provision of running exercise. Or there was overcrowding. There was even use of vaccination in some cases. There was dosage with common chemical tonics – and so on.

I was always able to tell the dissatisfied with absolute truth, and with witnesses available wherever I had raised my own animals by my own method in many lands – dogs, horses, goats, wild birds, bees – that they had known excellent health, good temperaments (even the bees!), resistance to disease, and enjoyed long life. The good health on Natural Rearing also included my two children, and the children of many other people. Finally, I wrote a book – *Natural Rearing of Children*, which Faber and Faber published in 1970. A later, revised edition was published in America by Schocken Books under the title of *Nature's Children*.

Finally, when you have raised your vitally alive and sensitive mature animals, please do exert the utmost vigilance to ensure that not one, neither puppy nor adult, is sold to a laboratory, there to endure lifelong imprisonment, terror and pain. The pain of unnatural diets and surgical woundings from which there is no escape is an outrage to God, who created dog to protect and companion man and never for such unspeakable treatment as vivisection, pharmacy tests, etc. *Take care!*

PART TWO

The Use of Herbs in Canine and Feline Ailments

6

Introduction to Herbal Medicine

In the following chapter there will be found in alphabetical order the common canine ailments and the herbs that relieve and cure them. If it is difficult for those who live in cities to go out and gather herbs, they can be obtained dried if need be from herbals shops, but those who can collect their own are referred to Chapter 10, where they are listed with their botanical names as well as a number of their popular (English) ones, so that with the aid of any standard work on wild flowers one can identify the plants to be quite sure that the right plant has been found. The botanical name is the same for all countries, so that readers should use a locally published book with illustrations as a guide. Most of the herbs used are common in England and America. For those who wish to use proprietary herbal products, see page 320.

Note: Faber and Faber have published a fully illustrated herbal of mine, which will add greatly to the identification of herbs, *The Illustrated Herbal Handbook for Everyone*, which contains nearly one hundred herb drawings by the well-known botanical artist, Heather Wood. These are truly expert drawings for teaching the identification of common herbs. This book, after many hardback editions, is now available as a paperback.

I have confined the ailments to the really common ones and to those that will respond to herbal treatment. I have not included in this book the vast number of canine diseases which are not readily curable and which are a direct result of long-term incorrect rearing – among them tuberculosis, cancer, and other morbid growths, also other chronic ailments which afflict the canine race – and most of which, if correct rearing were followed according to the laws of Nature, could certainly be avoided.

It might well be argued that if correct rearing methods were employed it surely ought to be both possible and simple to avoid disease altogether. But it must be appreciated that in the domesticated conditions under which most dogs are kept, really Natural Rearing methods are very difficult to follow. There is, for example, the flesh-foods question: the real flesh foods natural to the dog are mainly the smaller members of the animal kingdom such as rabbits, hares, sheep, goats, etc, all of which are seldom available in the meat stores of big towns, and especially not as food for dogs. The meat that is commonly fed to dogs is, instead, usually old cow or horse, and in many cases the flesh is that of diseased animals which have died as a result of their sickness, or indirectly as a result of the dosing with chemical drugs. Other factors which can undermine the health, even of the strongest and most correctly reared dog, are inclement weather, especially prolonged dampness – the dog being a sun-loving animal – and, further, infectious diseases carried by other dogs outside the breeder's own kennel, such as worms, skin parasites, and the several epidemic diseases. I should warn that some of the very worst are the vaccine-borne diseases because they are of *un*natural type and the normal dog defences are weak against them. Then, furthermore, there are the hereditary ailments and the general inheritance of ill health which is the direct result of the unnatural rearing methods of the last eighty years or so, when men first began to commercialize dog breeding and introduce cheap rearing methods, including devitalizing foods, in place of the natural ones. Such methods include overcrowding in unhygienic kennels, breeding from weakly stock, lack of exercise and, above all, unhealthy feeding. The standard diet used in breeding kennels up to seven or eight years ago – when the alarming state of canine health then forced breeders to adopt other feeding methods – was soaked white-flour biscuits with dried meat addition, the whole usually served up hot with greasy stock and occasional lumps of cooked flesh and bones. Such an unnatural diet and 100 per cent cooked is still in common use today, with the difference that canned meat is now the unnatural way of feeding flesh to dogs and cats, and it is worse than the cooked stuff because no one knows what types of flesh and 'by-products' go into these fancy-named cans.

I have, therefore, confined the ailments mainly to those which are quite common and which are likely to be met with, even in the best-managed kennels at times, especially because many conditions of the canine body which are described as diseases are in fact only cleansing efforts of the body, produced when the body has become internally unclean, or are simply glandular disturbances to be found in young stock around the time of puberty. It is a natural fact that the adolescent period in young stock should be accompanied by minor body disturbances, just as the same period in childen will often be accompanied by mild attacks of fevers which, as in the case of canine distemper, are easily and readily cured when *correctly* treated. But when incorrectly treated, by such methods as chemical and serum therapy, they can be turned into very serious conditions indeed, which well warrant the title of disease, and which can leave permanent sequelae, such as blindness, deafness, paralysis, nervous twitches, etc.

I have devoted much space to worm trouble, for more dogs are killed by dosing for worms than are ever killed by the worms themselves, and, further, severe suffering is frequently caused by the worm treatments in common use. Also in this chapter will be found the internal cleansing treatment, which is a necessary and basic part not only of worm removal but of the treatment of 90 per cent of canine ailments. (This begins on page 139.) It may seem questionable that one treatment should form the basis for the cure of such a number of diverse canine ailments, but it must not be forgotten that Nature herself provides only one basic treatment, no matter what the body disorder is – be it broken limb or serious fever – and that is curative fasting and the attendant release of all the healing powers which are natural to every living thing, from a tree to a human being. Anyone who has studied the ways of wild animals cannot fail to have observed that in sickness the animal completely abstains from food, taking itself away into some quite hiding place and there remaining until normal health is restored to the body. It is then that the healed animal seeks out remedial herbs to complete the cure, and it is interesting to observe how the different animals show preferences for different herbs. For instance, the dog is very partial to couch grass, mustard leaves, borage leaves and seaweed; the cat to couch grass and catmint; the wild deer to bilberries and broom-tops; the hare to sow-thistle; the cow to garlic leaves and watercress (when it can get the former – for farmers unwisely ban it).

I have given with the list of ailments instructions for the preparation of the herbal treatment. In every case the fresh-gathered herb should be used when possible, for it is only in the fresh state that all the wondrous healing powers contained in plant juices can be fully utilized; but, naturally, for the autumn and winter months it will be necessary to dry many of the herbs, although a number, such as rosemary, thyme, lavender, holly, southernwood and others are to a certain extent 'evergreen'. The herbs should be gathered when in full and fresh leaf, never when the leaf is fading; and for drying purposes a fine day is necessary, for if the herbs are gathered when rain- or dew-wet they will soon turn mouldy. To dry: they should be bunched in small quantities and hung in an airy place, or put in thin brown paper bags or in baskets, likewise in an airy place, or spread on sheets of paper (not newspaper) on tables or on fine mesh wire-netting and covered with cotton gauze to keep off dust. Never use plastic bags. All herbs when drying need frequent turning to ensure aeration and prevent formation of mould. In temperate climates mild heat can be used. Strong sunlight over-dries medicinal herbs, turns them yellow and destroys their medicinal values. A modern 'nasty' development in the herbal trade is electric drying of herbs, just as wheat is now mostly artificially dried for speed, instead of being allowed to mellow slowly outdoors in the stooks as in former times. Such quick-dried herbs are devoid of medicinal properties, therefore take care you are not sold such herbs for your dogs. The whole subject is dealt with completely in my full-length practical herbal handbooks – *The Complete Herbal Handbook for Farm and Stable* and *The Illustrated Herbal Handbook for Everyone*.

The dried herbs should be stored in strong-texture brown paper bags, the bags tightly tied at the neck. Place the tied bags in strong-texture cotton sacks (if not available then use new cotton pillow-cases). Tie the necks of bags and sacks tightly so that not the smallest insect can enter. Precautions must be taken not only against insects, but also against rodents, all of which are greedy for healthful medicinal herbs!

In the case of complete absence of sunlight at a time when it is necessary to dry the herbs, which is not unknown in parts of the world during the herb-drying season in late summer, a lukewarm oven should be used for the drying, keeping the door ajar. Herbs must be gathered fresh every year for drying, no matter how well they may have kept through the winter. Old herbs should not be retained; for that reason it is preferable for dog breeders to collect and dry their own herbs.

PREPARATION OF HERBS

STANDARD INFUSION The standard infusion used throughout this book is made from one large handful of the fresh herb (or two heaped tablespoons dry herb), cut up small if the herb has large leaves, prepared with a pint of cold water. Cover well, then simmer until near boiling point, do not boil. Then stand, off the heat, to brew for four hours. Do not strain. Pour into a clean jar, covering this with paper – not waxed – or cotton cloth against dust, etc. Make a fresh infusion every three days, two or less days in hot weather.

The average dose (throughout this book a cocker spaniel size dog is taken to represent average) is two level tablespoons of the infusion morning and night, and always at least thirty minutes before a meal. For the smaller and larger breeds, decrease or increase the dose accordingly. Unlike chemical canine remedies, all herbal medicines are harmless and therefore there is no fear of an overdose. That is why it is safe to give directions in handfuls; the need for extreme accuracy arises only when chemicals are used. Of course there are poisonous plants, but the herbalists should not deal in them. With the exception of opium poppy for urgent pain relief, they are unnecessary and dangerous, and I will not have my herbal work associated with them.

The best way of administering the infusions is from a plastic (thus supple) medicine bottle containing the correct dosage; the neck of the bottle is pressed into the near side of the dog's mouth and the bottle slowly emptied.

STRONG INFUSION When stronger infusions are required, the shredded herbs should be placed in an enamel pan with a half pint of *cold water* per handful of herbs (or more can be made at a time in proportion). Heat to boiling point, boil for no longer than three minutes, then set aside to brew for at least seven hours (it is preferable to leave overnight). Throughout the heating and steeping periods, keep tightly lidded to prevent escape of steam and volatile properties of herbs. After steeping, pour into a jar without straining, and cover to exclude dust, etc, but allow entry of air.

Most herbs for canine use need the standard infusion because cellulose is not easily digested by carnivorous animals. Human beings, cattle and horses can, of course, digest large quantities of raw herbs and obtain their medicinal benefits more easily. Dogs which are exceptionally difficult to dose must have their herbs very finely cut up or given in powder form, either mixed into balls with honey and pushed down the throat, or well blended with their food. The former is to be preferred, as the bitterness of many herbs when present in food may cause the dog to refuse the food.

I have evolved a method of giving herbs raw which has proved very effective. A concentrated herbal extract may be given in a small dosage, no more than one tablespoon twice daily for an average dog. To make the extract, squeeze a large handful of the fresh herbs into a ball, place on a grater for vegetables, bruise herb by rubbing well on grater with flat of fingers. When herb is pulpy, put it on a square of cheesecloth or cotton and add an extracting medium (raw milk or carrot juice, both particularly absorbent), two tablespoons of raw unboiled milk or juice of one medium carrot. When liquid and herb pulp are mixed, wring and twist cloth strongly. The extract retains all vitamins and cosmic forces unspoiled, and the flavour is strong and aromatic, far more so than with the general hot-water extraction method. Give by bottle.

PRACTICAL MEDICAL TREATMENTS

For the benefit of the novice, here is how to take a dog's temperature. Insert the mercury end of the thermometer in the anus (the opening of the lower bowel beneath the tail) so that all the mercury is covered. Keep the thermometer in that position for several minutes: then withdraw and read. Remember to shake the mercury well below the level of the normal temperature of 101·4° F before inserting. ('Normal' is different for every creature. A special dog thermometer can be bought at a chemist's.) High fever is indicated by a rise of temperature to 103° to 107° F. Wash the thermometer in cold water and pine fluid after use. If you suspect fever and have not got a thermometer, one can feel the inside of the ears with the hand. If temperature is normal they are merely slightly warm, in fever they are very hot.

Pulse: the normal beat per minute for the dog is 90 to 100 beats (for the cat, 110 to 120). To take the pulse beat, find an artery on the inside of the thigh, and press it with fingers on the bone; the pulse beats can then be felt and counted.

Eye diagnosis: this is very helpful as a health guide. When there is sickness, such as fever etc, the normally white areas of the eye are stained red, and the inner lids, both upper and lower, are red instead of a healthy pale pink. The pupils of the eyes also are changed, being dull looking.

To give a suppository: Do not first use Vaseline or glycerine as usually directed on the box wrapper; merely press the suppository into the anus and prevent the dog from expelling this for from three to five minutes.

To give an enema: a small bulb rectal syringe is required and about one and a half pints of warm water into which a teaspoon of witch hazel has been mixed (the witch hazel tones up the bowel walls); or lemon juice or common tea water can replace the witch hazel. Fill the syringe with the warm water and inject into the lower bowel slowly and steadily. Continue until all the fluid has entered the bowel, the animal's hind quarters being kept raised throughout. Then the dog will have a cleansing bowel evacuation. This type of enema does not take more than five minutes to carry out and is invaluable; as with herbal infusions, the quantity given is for an average dog – more or less fluid is required for larger or smaller breeds.

INTERNAL CLEANSING TREATMENT AND DIET

As the internal cleansing treatment diet, which I have evolved, forms the basis of most of the herbal cures for the ailments given in *Medicinal Herbs*, I am giving it in detail at the end of the chapter. The diet was created especially for canine distemper cure and, therefore, except in cases of fever ailments, can be considerably shortened. For instance, for a short course of internal cleansing, merely a two-day fast followed by a further two-day milk-honey fluid diet would be necessary; a return to normal diet could then be made.

Special Note: Treatment must begin with a fast of at least two days on water or honey-water only. Two to three days is usually sufficient to cure a straightforward fever case. During fasting all the body powers released from food digestion are concentrated on elimination of internal toxins, and therefore chances of curing the ailments are made more favourable. Urgency of toxin elimination supplies the important reason for use of a daily laxative when fasting or on the fluid diet of milk and honey. During long fasts if there is no natural bowel action, a warm-water enema is given. Until the temperature is normal and steady at normal, fasting *must* be continued. To

139

feed solid foods during a fever means complication of the ailment and often also fatal results.

When people do not want to put their animals on a total fast, honey and fruit juices such as grape or apple can be given. Honey and grapes feed the body more completely than meat, etc, at such times, and are easily digested.

FASTING In order to carry out with confidence this important part of the internal cleansing treatment, the principle of fasting must be understood. It is the natural instinct of all animals to fast when sick or wounded, because immediately all food is withheld, all the forces of the body are concentrated on fighting the disease or healing the wound, for the strength of the body is no longer being used up in the normal and continuous daily activity of food digestion, absorption, and elimination. Actually, when an animal is ill with fever, Nature discourages the intake of food by removing a desire for it and suspending senses of smell and taste: during acute fever, food digestion is checked almost totally.

If food is given forcibly at such times, poured into the mouth, severe bowel inflammation and thus diarrhoea are caused, and nerves also become inflamed. The chance, then, of the case making a satisfactory recovery is seriously diminished.

What actually happens during the fast? The body contrives to burn up the useless fat deposits, and until *all* fat is burnt up the vital tissues are left intact. As large amounts of body impurities are embedded in the fatty tissues of the average type of domestically reared dog, the body begins to be cleansed deeply, as the fat is oxidized; also the stomach and intestines, relieved of their usual tasks of dealing with food, can now concentrate on clearing away mucus deposits, worms and their ova (if present), toxins, etc. Therefore the

critical stage of the fever, which is usually prolonged in orthodox treatment, is speedily overcome in the natural cleansing-
fasting treatment, and after three or four days' fast all danger is
frequently over. If, however, the case under treatment is
already in an advanced stage through the owner's failure to
discover the early symptoms, and therefore the dog, though
sick, having been allowed to feed on heavy foods when its
temperature was raised above normal, a long fast is often
necessary, and in some cases a three-weeks' fast is required to
restore the temperature to normal. It should be stated here that
the dog's own inclination cannot always be relied upon. No
sick wild animal will eat food, but in the domestic dog natural
instinct has often long departed, and the urge of habit hunger
and routine meal times will often cause a sick dog to partake of
food; furthermore, a greedy desire for food when high fever is
present is frequently a serious sign of deranged nerves.

It has been well proved that any animal can fast for three
weeks (provided drinking water is available) without much
difficulty. The fur-seal male (bull) fasts for three *months* during
the breeding season. Also, when animals hibernate through
the winter months, they are carrying out a partial fast. In order
to understand more about fasting because of its importance in
my herbal veterinary work, I have carried out many experi-
mental fasts myself. The first three days are the most difficult
as the habit of desiring food at certain hours persists: but when
those days are past, the brain begins to feel unusually clear and
a feeling of extra well-being is experienced. It is this general
feeling of well-being which helps a very sick animal to make its
recovery from a disease. I have achieved many long fasts,
including one of sixteen days and one of three weeks.

The main difficulty in teaching fasting to the inexperienced
is the superstitious belief that a person or dog not having food
daily will starve. They think that one or two days without food
is the limit of human or animal endurance. And yet the yogis of

India will fast for many weeks without thinking it an event of importance. The students of the famed philosophe Pythagoras were required to fast their bodies for forty day before their brains were considered sufficiently purified t imbibe the profound teachings of this philosopher. Th theory of rapid starvation is discredited when one consider that, in order to starve, the skeleton condition must first b reached, and an animal cannot starve while an ounce of fa still remains on its body. And considering that a fever cas should be spending its time resting undisturbed in an eve temperature, with access to as much fresh drinking water a desired, very little expenditure of energy is needed and it normal fat supplies will last several weeks.

Dr Herbert M. Shelton writes knowledgeably concernin fasting and the lesson to be learned from animals.

Domestic cattle may often be found suffering from som chronic disease. Such animals invariably consume less foo than the normal animal. Every farmer knows that when cow, a horse, or hog, or sheep, etc, persistently refuse food, or day after day consumes much less than normally there is something wrong with the animal.

Dr Felix Oswald states: 'Serious sickness prompts al animals to fast. Wounded deer will retire to some seclude den and starve for weeks together.'

Dr Edwin Liek, a noted surgeon, endorses fasting, an observes that 'small children and animals, guided by an infal lible instinct, limit to the utmost their intake of food if the are sick or injured'. He describes the instinctive fasting o three of his dogs. One was run over, suffering internal injur ies and broken ribs; the second ate a quantity of rat poison the third lost an eye in a fight. All three fasted and recovered apart from eye replacement.

Professor Edmond Bordeaux Szekely has told me that onc

142

when his great hunting cat, Arriman, who used to catch and eat rattlesnakes, was bitten in the foot by one of those snakes, the cat allowed no one to touch him. He went to a swift-running stream, where he selected and ate quantities of a grass growing by it; he kept his injured foot deep in the water for one entire day and night with no other food. He fully recovered. Animals are usually their own best doctors. Asclepius, the Greek patron saint of medicine, always taught that dogs are the most clever of the creatures because they know best what wild weeds to select and eat to cure all canine ailments.

Physiologists have persistently ignored those cases where dogs have voluntarily fasted for ten or twenty-eight or more days when suffering from broken bones or internal injuries. Here is an action invariably pursued by Nature which they persist in refusing to investigate. The enforced fasting of animals during modern warfare when trapped in bombed buildings has given many remarkable examples, cases having survived after as long as one month without food *or* water. Sheep have been buried for months in snowdrifts and have been rescued alive: but they have been able to eat the snow for water.

Those who have had no experience of fasting claim that it weakens the body. But the first weakness of fasting is merely due to habit hunger and passes after the first few days. Food does not give strength during fever. I have seen too many examples of the 'three-hourly feeds' orthodox treatment, which remove all doubt as to which treatment is correct, the natural or the unnatural. The feeding-during-fever cases are generally skeleton thin and foul-smelling internally, their bodies jerking with chorea, racked with fits, and many blinded with excessive eye discharges.

Then it is further often stated that without food during fever the blood is weakened. That such a statement is unscientific is demonstrated by the fact that laboratory tests of the blood of fasting cases, made before, during, and after the conclusion of the fast, show that the number of the vital red blood corpuscles is considerably *increased* by the fast.

I cannot over-emphasize that the giving of food to an animal with a high temperature is positively and undeniably the cause of most of the nervous complications found in canine distemper, for example. Of the hundreds of fever cases sent to me for treatment, only a very few cases developed mental symptoms, and each of them had reached me in a very advanced stage of the disease; the damage to the nervous system had been caused already.

The good quality of the drinking water is of utmost import-ance during long fasting, and in most large cities, where the water supply is heavily chlorinated, it is advisable to buy bottled spring water, usually obtainable from chemists. Do not buy unnatural distilled water or bottled water 'purified' by unnatural methods. Rain-water is good if collected in clean country air.

Of importance is the daily cleansing of the bowels. If diarrhoea is present or not, a daily laxative is still needed during fasting to cleanse away mucus and other impurities being loosened. Senna pods are best (for preparation, see Internal Cleansing Diet). In lengthy fasting, give a rectal enema (see directions, page 138).

The fast must be continued while the temperature is around 102·6° F or above, food not being permitted until the temperature has remained steady around 101·4° F for at least four days. If the fever should return when the second, or feeding, stage of the treatment is in progress, this event being indicated by a sudden abrupt rise of temperature to around 103° F or above, then the fast must be followed again. Such relapses are not common, but the fact that they do occur occasionally should not be ignored. Note that the normal

emperature of young puppies is often 102° F, and higher for
he excitable ones who have a normal temperature of around
102·8° F. It is seldom necessary to fast a young puppy longer
han two to four days before a cure of fever symptoms or
dysentery is obtained. Watered milk with honey is permiss-
ble for young puppies.

Throughout the fasting stage pure honey can be given, and
in exhaustion give fresh, not bottled, canned or packeted
juice of fresh grapes or apples or pomegranates. Two des-
sertspoonfuls at usual meal times, when food would have
been given if the case was not being fasted, are an average
dose for a medium size dog.

Herbal tablets of powerful antiseptic herbs, with a garlic
base, should be given morning and night, two three-grain
tablets being an average dose each time. Their use is highly
important. If these are not available, then rosemary herb, as
sold in tins or packets at grocery stores, should be brewed by
the standard method, and into this, when cold, should be
crushed some garlic juice, using a juice extractor or mincing
the garlic and pressing it through muslin – a small teaspoon
of garlic to one dessertspoon of rosemary for an average size
dog. *Note:* average size means spaniel.

Internal Cleansing Diet (for fever cases)

The amounts given here are for an average size dog. Decrease
or increase according to size of the individual breed.

First day Three meals per day of tepid water only. One
teaspoon of pure lemon juice can be added per meal. Do not
use bottled or synthetic lemon juice.

Two herbal compound tablets or garlic plant, for internal
disinfecting, morning and night throughout this treatment.
Some form of laxative, preferably senna pods (Alexandria

type), three pods soaked seven hours in two tablespoons col
water, with a pinch of powdered ginger added, is average
Do not give oil laxatives. Give this senna at night.

Second day Repeat first day, including laxative at night.

Third day Three meals per day of honey and water (on
heaped teaspoon of honey to one cup of tepid water). Als
fresh water to drink. Or herbal teas can be used instead of
plain water (such herbs as sage, thyme, marjoram). Add
sprig of antiseptic southernwood to the tea herbs, if obtair
able. (See Standard Infusion, page 136.) Southernwood
very bitter so use very little. Laxative at night.

Fourth day Repeat third day. Laxative.

Fifth day Repeat third day. Laxative.

Sixth day Repeat third day. Provided the temperature is no
normal, around 101·4° F, the honey-water can now k
replaced by three small meals daily of unboiled cow's d
goat's milk, preferably unpasteurized, of course, as he
treatment destroys the healing properties of milk. Pasteu
ized milk may have to be used if no other is available. Do no
give other milks such as canned, long-life, etc.

Now give Natural Rearing vegetable tablets, two tablets pe
day. If tablets are not available, give minced green sala
vegetables, such as dandelion, watercress, turnip, and mu
tard greens, one dessertspoon at meal times. Suggested time
for meals, 8 a.m., 12 noon, 6 p.m. Laxative to be discor
tinued.

Seventh day Repeat sixth day.

Eighth day Repeat sixth day, but alter evening meal k
adding to the milk-honey one handful of flaked cereal, barle
preferably; otherwise, use oats.

Ninth day Repeat eighth day, increasing cereal to two handfuls.

Tenth day Repeat eighth day, but now increase cereal to an ample feed. Sprinkle the cereal with powdered or flaked natural wheat germ, approximately one tablespoon. A few raisins, cut up small, can be added.

Eleventh day Repeat tenth day.

Twelfth day Cease 8 a.m. meal and replace midday meal with one cup of steamed fish plus a sprinkle of flaked oats and wheat germ.

Thirteenth day Repeat twelfth day.

Fourteenth day Repeat thirteenth day.

Fifteenth day Repeat first day, i.e. water fast, to rest and recleanse the internal organs.

Sixteenth day Repeat twelfth day, but now add other cereals to the barley-milk feed; preferably whole-grain oats, rye, etc. A little whole-grain bread or some whole-grain biscuits can be fed now.

The dog should now be ready to go on to the normal Natural Rearing diet (see Chapter 1, page 49).

An important additional food is now the oxygen obtained only through outdoor running exercise.

Note: the carrying-out of the internal cleansing diet is left to the discretion of the person in charge of the sick dog or cat. It should always be remembered that the diet is dependent on the temperature, and the presence of any fever should always be treated by fasting. Also great care must be taken in the ending of the fast. No more than stated quantities of solid foods given in the diet are permitted. To allow a dog to gorge itself after a long fast on fluids could have fatal results. The fasting must be ended carefully and gently, only very small amounts of solid foods being given for the first few days.

Fruit juices, especially lemon, apple, blackcurrant, and grape, are permitted during fasting. But do not give orange or tomato, neither being beneficial foods for sick dogs.

A TONIC PILL   Chamomile one ounce, thyme one ounce, rue half ounce, cloves quarter ounce, ginger quarter ounce (all in powder form). Mix well and then roll into a solid mass, binding with thick honey, or thick palm oil, and wheaten or oat flour. Divide into pills which the animal can swallow (one to two teaspoons dosage) and give as required. Store in a glass jar in a cool place or refrigerator.

7

Ailments and their Treatments
(in Alphabetical Order)

Note: for Standard Infusion and Strong Infusion, see instructions, Chapter 6, Preparation of Herbs, p. 136. Unless otherwise stated, the amounts of all herbs prescribed in the treatments are: one handful of fresh or two tablespoons dry herbs to one pint of water.

ALL THE TREATMENTS ARE SUITABLE FOR CATS.

ABRASION   Caused usually through biting at an itching part, especially in skin diseases, or can be caused through ill-fitting collar, or from an accident which tears off the hair.

Treatment Make an infusion of young leaves of blackberry and apply externally twice daily; a little witch hazel extract can be added with advantage: a quarter teaspoon witch hazel to every tablespoon of the blackberry infusion. Elder flowers and leaves of rosemary can be used instead. No greasy ointments should be used: such dressings soften the tissues and retard the cure.

ABSCESS   Found on any part of the body and commonly between the toes, where they are called interdigital cysts.

Treatment Fomentations with blackberry or elder infusion, keeping the lotion hot during application. Do not add witch hazel now, as astringent is not required. An excellent poultice can be made by macerating three cloves of garlic root, or the heart of an onion. Stir this into two ounces of castor oil. Place the mixture in a small jar or tin with fairly loose cover, then place the jar in a pan of cold water to reach half-way up the jar, and bring the pan of cold water to a slow boil, heating the jar until the garlic or onion turns quite soft in the oil. Then wring out a piece of cotton in hot water, pour the hot lotion on to the hot cotton (but not too hot) and bind over the abscess, using as a wrapping a piece of towelling that is dry and also hot.

An excellent alternative poultice is boiled turnip or parsnip, spread on cotton, as with the garlic-castor treatment.

ANAL GLANDS TROUBLE Dogs rarely suffer from internal piles, but are quite commonly affected with a form of external piles known as anal glands trouble. The anus becomes swollen and surrounded with a number of small lumps which discharge blood when pressed. Haemorrhoids can also occur. Sufferers are usually overfed pets; also many of the toy breeds. The trouble would not occur if dogs were fed a natural diet which always included sufficient roughage.

Treatment Dosing with a brew of dandelion (leaves and/or flowers); also, soak fenugreek seeds in warm water, two tablespoons to one cup or more, for twenty-four hours, then give the liquid as a drink, and feed the seeds mixed into the cereal feed. Give linseed tea, strong infusion; also apply the tea externally. In severe cases, make suppositories from pulped, raw dock leaves and insert in the anus. Also apply diluted witch hazel.

ANAEMIA Usually caused through incorrect diet or lack of sunlight, or constipation.

Treatment Medicine of any of the black fruits, such as bramble, bilberry, elderberry, or grape, when in season given crushed into the cereal feed or as a standard infusion. Two tablespoons of infusion for an average size dog. Add a teaspoon of honey to every tablespoon of herbal infusion. When all the black fruits are out of season, nettle can be used; this herb contains natural iron at its best, very different from chemical iron, which is constipating and aggravates anaemia. Feed also raw eggs, seaweed, molasses, parsley.

APPETITE, LOSS OF   Loss of appetite is an unfailing sign of toxic condition in the stomach or intestines, or both. Many dogs live almost their entire lives in such a state, picking at their food instead of devouring it in the manner of a healthy dog; they are described as 'bad-doers', but they are merely internally clogged and filthy, or they may be deprived of normal free-running exercise, essential to maintain good health.

Treatment   Internal dosing with an infusion of peppermint, using the flowers and small stalks in addition to the leaves, if available. Cress seed, sown out of doors or indoors and cultivated until a plant of three inches high with parsley-like leaves is produced, and given finely shredded with the meat feed, is an excellent appetite restorer. Grated raw apple is also good. A course of internal cleansing, to purify the entire digestive tract, is an essential part of the treatment; the fasting period should be anywhere from three to seven days or until the dog shows a really keen desire for any food offered to it. Careful dieting on Natural Rearing lines (see normal diet, Chapter 1) is a further essential, in order to keep the digestive tract clean and healthy once it has been cleansed through the fasting treatment. Whenever a dog leaves any food in the feeding-dish, that food should be removed immediately and the dog kept without until the next meal time. Giving food snacks in between the two meals per day permitted is fatal to good appetite and sound health. Plenty of running exercise should also form a part of the treatment. Charcoal tablets are an excellent appetite restorative; and minced-up raw celery. Give also NR Health Cakes (Daily Health) daily.

Note: Exception to the feeding rule is the greyhound breed. Afghans, salukis, etc, are often slow eaters; their meals have to stay with them several hours, sometimes overnight.

ARTHRITIS   This ailment once rare in the dog has become quite common. Joints often become knobby and gait stiffens. Damp, sunless rearing, also lack of adequate exercise, all encourage arthritis, even though an over-acid diet is the chief cause.

Treatment   Internal dosing with rosemary brew; also feed chopped, raw parsley and comfrey leaves mixed in with the meat. Comfrey is often called the 'arthritic herb'. Boiled nettles are also curative. Externally massage the area with a lotion of four tablespoons olive oil, one part linseed oil, to which add a half teaspoon eucalyptus oil. Sunflower oil is also good, used in place of the linseed. Also helpful is Vick's Vapo-Rub.

ASTHMA   Flat-nosed breeds, such as Pekinese, pugs and bull-dogs, are more prone to this trouble. But if dogs or bitches of any breed become very obese, they are prone to asthma. The common wayside herb of sticky foliage, elecampane, is the specific cure for this trouble. The flowers of chrysanthemum are also good. Keep the animal on a laxative diet when attacks are severe. Give plenty of fresh air.

Treatment   Make a strong brew of elecampane (whole herb) and give a tablespoon morning and night, sweetened with honey. Also boil some elecampane, remove from the heat and hold the dog's face over the herbal steam, placing a cloth over its head, to serve as an inhalation. (For alternative inhalations, see Pneumonia.) In addition, pound up four chrysanthemum flowers per day for an average size dog, and make into pills with honey and flour.

BAD BREATH Very common in old dogs, but also in young dogs of the toy breeds, this is generally due to food decomposition and to constipation; in old dogs bad teeth may be responsible.

Treatment Internal dosing with an infusion of rosemary leaves, flowers, or both; the mouth and teeth can also be washed with some of the infusion. A short course of internal cleansing is necessary, followed by corrective dieting. If dogs were fed correctly, according to the laws of Nature, bad breath would never occur, and dogs would keep their teeth in good condition up to the time of their death, no matter how great their age. Regular cleansing, fasting, and correct feeding are especially necessary in the rearing of the toy breeds; their stomachs and intestines are so minute, regular 'resting' is essential, and what little food is fed to them must be of the highest possible quality; using rye as half of the cereal ration would benefit the toy breeds. In general, in bad breath, the inclusion in the diet of shredded dried fruits would benefit all breeds; dried fruits sweeten the stomach and digestive tract and are gently laxative. It is possible to obtain charcoal tablets from most chemists: they will purify the entire digestive tract. Give also raw, finely minced carrot, parsley and mint.

BALDNESS This trouble is especially prevalent among certain breeds, especially the dachshund, chow and Pekinese, and is referred to later under the heading of Mange. However, there is another less serious state of baldness which affects many of the smooth-coated breeds, especially when they are in a state of low health; for example, bitches after the rearing of a litter for which correct dietary preparation had not been made, distemper after-effects, nerve disorders, etc. The condition can be cleared up quickly through corrective diet and external herbal washes.

Treatment A corrective raw-foods diet, especially rich in fresh raw meat, with a daily dosage of raw chopped dandelion leaves combined with the meat (the copper content of dandelion leaves being especially effective in the treatment); give daily powdered seaweed. Exposure to all possible sunlight. Washes of an infusion of rosemary leaves or marigold flowers, both equally excellent. The bald areas should be bathed daily with the brew of rosemary or marigold. A brew made from daffodil leaves is an old gypsy remedy for baldness and falling hair. Rub the resultant liquid into the affected areas several times a day. Castor oil applied externally, well massaged into the bare areas, has proved excellent and is extra effective when a few drops of oil of eucalyptus are added.

BITES (See also Bleeding) The dog is a pack animal and asserts itself by biting to protect its rights so most dogs are bitten at some time by their fellow canines. They also suffer from bites of insects and snakes.

Treatment *Dog Bites:* bathe the area with a strong brew of rosemary herb. A speedier remedy, and proved effective for bites and all kinds of wound, is to pour wine over the wound, ordinary white or red wine is best. If bites are deep treat as for Bleeding.

Insect Bites: there are many instant remedies well proved as effective. Immediate application of any of the following remedies – vinegar of any kind; juice pressed from a fresh lemon or from garlic cloves; whitewash paste, but remove after an hour as it burns the skin. Follow on treatment with a strong brew of rosemary. To help protect against harmful biting insects such as mosquitoes and fleas (alas, there is no total protection), spray, using a puffer spray with fine holes, all hairless parts of the dog with insect repellent herbal powder, morning and night. Apply the powder particularly to the genitals, under the tail, the inner thighs and armpits. I so often go into mosquito-infested areas in the course of my herbal work and am so thankful I can protect my dogs in this way. When no herbal powder is available, spraying with talcum powder (as strongly scented as possible) will also protect from insect bites and is advised by vets. That very serious ailment lachmanias, carried by an insect of a lesser mosquito type and a killer in the Middle East and Mediterranean areas, can also be prevented by internal and external treatment with bitter herbs. Internal dosing with cayenne pepper is also effective.

It is a good idea, before mosquito-time, to take dogs indoors, if possible; put them in their kennels or in the house and puff-spray bitter mosquito repellent herbs, in fine powder form, on them – wormwood, southernwood, rue, pennyroyal, rosemary – such as used to deter fleas. Apply a spot of eucalyptus, or spirit of eucalyptus, on top of their heads, on ears, down the spine and tail, using a piece of wet cotton.

Mosquitoes dislike smoke, so make a smoky fire outdoors in the evenings; burn especially thuja pine because mosquitoes hate it. Pyrethrum burning coils are also useful: they are non-chemical but nevertheless slightly toxic. As a further precaution make sure there is no stagnant water near the house to furnish breeding places for the pests. Even wet nylon bags, litter and old cartons can provide breeding places.

Encourage bats to visit one's garden; they are the most skilled of mosquito and midge killers. The birds such as swallows and swifts visit gardens in the evening to catch flies and mosquitoes. Encourage them by providing natural quiet at that time of day.

Poisonous Bites (from such as scorpions and snakes): treatment must be immediate. First suck out and then spit out any of the poison which can be taken from around the bite; then apply anti-poison herbs such as, and particularly, rue, garlic and wormwood. These are best when infused in oil, either by strong sunheat or by fire-heat using a double heater and a process of slow extraction. I always keep in readiness a solution in oil of Herbal Protection powder, which contains both rosemary and wormwood as well as other effective herbs. The dog should be fasted for a day and given laxative at night. Make pills of two teaspoons each of rue, wormwood and garlic, minced fine and bound with thick honey and flour. Or give NR Herbal Compound tablets, which contain all three herbs among others.

While in Greece, my daughter's saluki bitch was bitten in the left foot by a yellow scorpion and was hysterical from the pain. I at once applied the herbal oil and maintained frequent applications. I also dosed her internally with Herbal Compound tablets and recovery was remarkably swift. We had visiting us an Austrian student, whose parents were both doctors, and he declared that never in his life had he seen anything cure so quickly as those herbs I had used. An apparently dying dog at night, by the following morning she was running around totally well.

Quick emergency treatments used by peasant people when

herbs are not available, and when scorpions or snakes have been identified as the biters, are garlic or lemon juice (freshly squeezed, not synthetic) or ammonia. Hot, not cold, cloths are applied at frequent intervals.

I would not personally use orthodox treatment, which is an antidote of the venom of the animal or insect concerned, but I would not advise against its use for others. Such treatments have saved life and there may not be anything else available as a cure.

But I do advise against meddlesome anti-tetanus injections, which nowadays are used for the most trivial bites and wounds. Nor would I accept rabies injections if I or any of my dogs were bitten by a rabid dog, but again this is a personal opinion: I would use herbal treatments and fasting.

BLADDER TROUBLES (stone and gravel, also irritability and inflammation) Bladder and kidney disorders are extremely common in the modern dog, the latter certainly being hereditary to a large extent, although they are also readily caused through the same factors responsible for the majority of canine ailments: incorrect and unnatural rearing. Chlorinated tap water is another cause.

Treatment Internal dosing with an infusion of the root of couch grass; this infusion is prepared differently from the standard method, the herb having to be simmered a full quarter-hour in the water. First, well bruise the root, then take two ounces of the root, over which pour three-quarters of a pint of boiling water, simmer gently until only a half pint of the liquid remains; then brew and prepare in the usual way; couch grass root possesses remarkable stone-dissolving properties.

Another excellent remedy is young birch leaves, infused in the standard way. A course of internal cleansing is recommended; and in the diet the addition of very finely shredded parsley and carrot added to the meat feed; the use of barley in place of the usual wheat cereal is very helpful (the barley must be whole grain, never 'pearl' or 'patent' barley, both being unnatural acid-producing foods). Pure honey gives remarkable aid and relief in bladder and kidney disorders, and is best given with the cereal feed. Operations for the removal of stone should never be resorted to until natural treatment has been given a thorough trial. Remarkable results have been obtained in the treatment of bladder and kidney disorders by the above method. The Rivaway Kennels, Beeston, Nottinghamshire, report:

> We had a Chow dog very ill with kidney trouble; the veterinary surgeon said he was a hopeless case, incurable. That is more than eighteen months ago; he is now a most beautiful dog (his photograph is in *Our Dogs Annual*). We gave him parsley water three times a day, and milk and barley water sweetened with honey. When his appetite came back, chopped parsley was added to his feed. He still has parsley and so do all the others.

BLEEDING OF WOUNDS When there is a great amount of bleeding from a wound, the blood outflow should be controlled and the torn flesh soothed by the application of a healing herb infusion. In all but the very deep-seated wounds there should be no bandaging, for the action of the dog's tongue in keeping the wound moist and breaking up the pus formations is alone a most remarkable healing process; bandaging would prevent the dog from making use of it. The formation of pus should never cause worry; that is Nature's own method of keeping the wound open and moist, for if a wound were to become sealed up at too early a stage in the healing process, any external impurities which may have found their way into the body tissue at the time of the wounding are then encouraged to set up poisoning, which may prove serious enough to cause death. In very deep-seated wounds the method of the great Spanish surgeon, Trueta, as practised with such success in the Spanish Civil War, should be followed. The wound should be laid freely open, all damaged tissue cut cleanly away so that the wound is left well exposed. Then pack the wound round with damp cotton wool and immobilize by making a loosely fitting plaster-of-Paris jacket to cover the injured part; note carefully the instruction 'loosely fitting'. The deep wound is then left to the healing powers of Nature; the formation of pus keeps the wound open and moist until the internal tissues are well healed.

How very different from the artificial methods of chemical medicine, so popular until Surgeon Trueta's remarkable results in wound healing caused his method to be adopted by large numbers of doctors in place of the orthodox one, with its harmful dry gauze placed over the raw wounds, the frequent scraping away of all pus formations, and the application of chemical disinfectants: the Trueta method has revealed the harm done in medicine, in my opinion, by Pasteur's friend Joseph Lister, the pioneer of chemical disinfectant wound dressings.

Spider webs (cobwebs) are a well-known primitive method of plugging deep wounds because they possess adhesive properties (swallows use them for binding their mud nests). They must be taken from clean places and shaken to remove any dust, etc. Fresh leaves of geranium, nasturtium, vine, castor oil, mallow (when tender) placed on wounds and held in place by a damp cotton bandage have great healing powers. Rinse leaves before use.

Treatment Herbal treatment to control the flow of blood from a severe wound, and to soothe and cleanse the injured tissues, is provided by a strong infusion of rosemary or the meadowsweet plant, both flowers and leaves being used, or hyssop. The infusion can be used both externally and internally; if given internally it strengthens the tissue-repairing powers of the body. If the wound is very deep and it is therefore necessary to use the Trueta method, an excellent natural dressing for packing around the wound beneath the plaster covering is sphagnum moss. This moss is a remarkable herb: it grows in damp places, in many parts of the world. The chief propery of sphagnum moss is its natural iodine content. It would not be out of place here to warn against the use of artificial chemical iodine, once the most-boosted wound and bruise treatment of the orthodox medical profession. In the words of one of the great pioneers of natural healing, Dr Lindlahr, 'the action of chemical iodine on living tissue is that of a mummifying agent, and prevents all normal healing, while encouraging the growth of excessively coarse scar tissue'. The same can be said for almost all of the chemical disinfectants. Another important treatment rule is: if the wounds are severe, and loss of blood considerable, a fast of one to several days is very necessary: most animals will voluntarily refrain from eating when severely wounded. At such times all of the internal forces of the body are required for cleansing, repair, and healing: they must not be wasted on food digestion. Dosage with leaf-extract tablets is most beneficial. For this green 'blood' of plant leaves does build red corpuscles and makes new blood in a far more natural way than transfusions of animal blood – as well as having none of the toxins that such blood must invariably contain.

Miss Sheelagh Seale, of the Ballykelly Irish Wolfhounds and Deerhounds, Avoca, Eire, reported the rapid recovery from severe wounds of a deerhound bitch. The bitch was badly bitten in a fight, and it was thought that she would die of her wounds. To quote Miss Seale:

When the vet left after seeing her for the first time, he said that my only hope to pull her through was sulphonamide drugs. The sulphonamides, of course, were *not* given. And when the vet came five days later the herbal treatment had produced the usual great results, and he was surprised to find the bitch so well, and all her wounds quite clean and healing up. The bitch has quite recovered now.

On my world travels I have usually had an Afghan hound with me as a guard. Being swift-running and wild-natured dogs, they have had their fair share of physical accidents, especially deep wounds from sharp-pointed desert vegetation, sharp rocks, etc. I have never stitched any of their wounds, despite some of them being deep enough to insert a hand fully inside. I have only relied on the healing and antiseptic powers of rosemary as a wound lotion (and, when this was not obtainable, using the more common plantain). I have also healed the torn udders of cows, leaking milk badly, by using rosemary for bathing, and plugging wounds with witch hazel on cotton, and also with clean (not dusty) spiderwebs.

In areas where flies are a problem, the protection of wounds by green leaves (already described) is very useful and curative. I have even cured severe gangrene in this way. Change the leaves every four hours. They will be very hot and wilt from the heat taken from the wound.

BREAST TUMOURS (also other tumours) Tumours in the milk glands area sometimes develop in bitches, and can be caused by blows, or merely from general ill health. Disordered glandular functions and constipation are also common causes, and an internal cleansing treatment, using the very solvent remedy grape juice, will often effect a cure. The tendrils and leaves of grape vine (from unsprayed vines), also fresh grape juice, have been used very effectively by the Arabs as an internal and external cure for tumours. The Mexican peasants use nopal cactus leaves, freed from prickles, in a way similar to the grape cure. Violet leaves have won fame with powers of dissolving tumorous and other growths. There is recorded the case of Lady Margaret Marsham, whose throat was completely blocked by a malignant growth, and which growth was entirely dissolved through the use of violet leaves. The violet-leaf infusion should both be given internally – two tablespoons morning and night – and applied externally – massaging the area of the tumour with the infusion on rising and retiring. Red clover, the leaves and flowers, or merely the leaves, can replace the violet leaves for both internal and external use when there is difficulty in obtaining the latter. Garlic and turnip also dissolve tumours, and rock-rose is valuable internally. Aloe vera, the internal pulp from sliced leaves, is also curative.

In severe cases, poultices made from fresh goosegrass and applied to the affected area are also very helpful. (The goosegrass, like sphagnum moss, is rich in natural iodine.) Since the earlier editions of *Medicinal Herbs*, I have been lent back copies of that excellent journal, *The Countryman*, in which the effect of violet brew was discussed in detail in the correspondence columns in relation to the cure of tumours. Among much interesting information given is the fact that the native doctors of Puerto Rico use a local violet (*Viola odorata*) to cure mild cancer of the stomach. The Turks recommend large quantities of watercress, to be eaten daily, and cures have been achieved by this simple treatment. For canine use, of course, all plant matter – violet, cresses, etc – would have to be given in a finely minced form to be digestible.

BROKEN BONES   (See Limbs, fractures of)

BRONCHITIS   (See Pneumonia)

BURNS   (See Scalds)

CANCER   (See also Breast Tumours) This terrible, killing disease was in former times almost unknown to the dog and the other carnivores. As chances of cure, even with herbs, are very slight, I am not going to suggest a herbal cure to prolong a disease usually so painful, and fatal. Cancer is alarmingly on the increase among domestic dogs and cats. Thousands of these loyal animals die every year after great suffering. Leukaemia, blood cancer, is now one of the most prevalent forms. Poisoning of the bloodstream by modern air pollution is a common reason, so is over-vaccination.

Prevention   depends upon Natural Rearing on pure natural foods similar to what the carnivores and felines eat in the wild; also provision of sufficient exercise.

CANKER   Canker of the ear is common to the domestic dog, especially to the breeds with long ear flaps which exclude air. One form of canker can be treated only by surgery; this is when heredity over-narrows the ear passage, excluding all normal air; a false air duct has then to be made by surgery. Long ears, especially, should be cleansed daily with standard rosemary infusion, three parts, and one part witch hazel extract. Keep inner ear flaps clean, using diluted witch hazel.

Treatment   Numerous cases have been cured by simple use of raw lemon juice, one-half teaspoon of the juice diluted with one and a half dessertspoons warm water. If the canker is simple, and not caused by an ear parasite called ear mite, it will merely be necessary to cleanse the ears daily, internally, with an infusion of horehound, or one made from equal quantities of violet leaves and wild poppy leaves or flowers.

The ears can then be further cleansed with witch hazel extract to remove the waxy deposits, and finally dusted over with finely powdered oatmeal; or the witch hazel could be used with the horehound or violet-poppy infusion, i.e. to one teaspoon of the infusion, four drops of witch hazel may be added. To cleanse the ears: twist a swab of cotton wool around the end of a pair of long tweezers, dip into the lotion, and very gently clean out the ear, frequently changing the cotton wool; about one level teaspoon of the lotion can then be dropped into each ear every morning, and well massaged, the ear being cleaned out with the tweezers and *dry* cotton wool in the evening. I have seen this lotion cure ears which were entirely blocked with the dark matter found in neglected or incorrectly treated ear canker.

In the form of canker caused by a small insect parasite, some insecticidal agent must be used. Powdered bitter herbs, of the kind described in the home remedies in this book, a heaped teaspoon to a cup of hot water. (Wormwood/southernwood alone could be used.) Add some spice cloves. Brew the lotion, add a few drops of oil of eucalyptus (as much as the case will tolerate, as it stings), use morning and night. Pour a teaspoon of brew into each ear, then swab out with cotton wool, as described above.

Note: Ears are highly sensitive so internal cleansing with cotton swabs on tweezers must be very gentle, the cotton held between the blades and then twisted around. Use new swabs for each ear.

A short course of internal cleansing would improve the general health of the dog, which is often impaired when canker is present. An infusion of garden thyme can also be given internally as a tonic, and will thus soothe the inflamed nerves of the ear and head through internal influence.

Mrs N. Howard, the Chastletown gundog breeder,

Wolverhampton, wrote me concerning two springer spaniel stud dogs which had been suffering for a long time from very severe ear canker, which had been unsuccessfully treated by three different veterinary surgeons. In her first letter, Mrs Howard told me that the condition of the dogs' ears was so bad she thought that she would have to have them both destroyed. However, internal cleansing was suggested to her, in addition to the external treatment with herbs. The ears of both dogs were entirely cured and the dogs themselves became very healthy.

Mrs Leslie Harrison, of Tarporley, Cheshire, famous for her pedigree goats and borzois, reported to me: 'A spaniel condemned by a foremost North-of-England vet as having incurable ear canker is now rising thirteen years and completely cured by your herbal treatment and so full of life it is wonderful to see him.'

CATARACT AND EYE ULCERS AND AILMENTS Vitamin A is an important preventative of eye infections. To ensure its presence in the daily diet, raw, green, minced vegetables should be given. Vitamin A is also present in animal fats such as unrefined cod-liver oil, halibut oil, meat fats, nut fats and whole, raw milk. Further, in raw and cooked carrots and sunlight. However, note that meat fat and cod-liver oil are often nowadays unhealthy toxic wastes.

Treatment Bathing the eye with an infusion of the leaves and flowers of the greater celandine, favourite eye remedy of the famed herbalist of ancient times, Culpeper. The eyes should be bathed twice daily with the celandine infusion which is to be used externally only. A course of internal cleansing should also be followed, to strengthen the whole body and thus the eyes also.

A strong infusion of flowers of rue or leaves of sage is used by Spanish peasants with much success. Use the same way as greater celandine. A standard infusion of either rosemary, chickweed, elder, mallow flowers, or dock leaves, all are good for inflamed eyes, as also is raw cucumber juice squeezed into the eyes and, further, cold Indian or China tea with the addition of a few drops of honey can be used with benefit for bathing them.

CHOREA Although nearly always a sequela of wrongly treated distemper, chorea sometimes occurs as a separate ailment. It is one of the most readily curable of the canine nervous ailments, the treatment given here having produced excellent results, healing many cases condemned as incurable by orthodox treatment. The only fatality is when the important motor nerve is affected.

Treatment An infusion of skullcap herb, the whole plant. Two tablespoons three times daily. Other internal chorea aids are: poppy seed heads, rue, rosemary, peony root, vervain, cayenne pepper (this pepper given as *tabasco* sauce, or compressed into tablets to be given morning and night). Also pomegranate juice is helpful, the pomegranates to be sliced across like lemons for squeezing.

For external treatment, make an infusion of lavender, marjoram, or thyme, or an infusion of all three; apply hot to the twitching areas. Give a course of internal cleansing treatment as a general nerve tonic. Feed as an extra, minced lettuce leaves and garden mint, minced rose hips – all are sedative to the nerves – also grape juice, fresh or bottled.

CONSTIPATION Just as correct diet is the only preventative of constipation, so likewise corrective dieting is the only cure for the ailment. No amount of dosing with chemical laxatives will effect a cure: such drastic dosing will only aggravate the trouble by weakening yet further the intestinal muscles, the healthy condition of which is essential for the regular and complete evacuation of waste matter from the body. In constipation, the toxins of the waste matter of the body, instead of being expelled daily through the bowel, are retained in the body and absorbed back into the bloodstream. It therefore cannot be wondered at that constipation is the root cause of a large number of canine ailments, from the lesser ones, such as eczema, to the acute ailments, such as cancer of the bowels, now becoming a common complaint.

Treatment As I have already said, the only curative treatment for constipation is through corrective diet, which will remove blocking toxic accumulations from the bowels, and will also restore to the intestinal muscles that natural strength which is necessary for the moving of the food residues down the bowel, and the complete expulsion of the bowel contents through the anus twice, or at least once, daily. The finest natural correctives of constipation, even in the case of the carnivorous dog, are fruits. Many dogs, if taught from puppyhood, will freely eat dried fruits with their cereal feed. Suitable dried fruits are figs, dates, raisins, and prunes – prunes being especially beneficial. Many dogs will eat fresh fruits and berries; they should be encouraged. Likewise, let them eat excreta of grass-fed animals. (See also notes on senna-pod laxatives, pp. 145–6). They also need ample fibre in the form of bran and whole-grain cereals. Desiccated coconut is helpful too.

COUGHING Coughing in dogs is generally a symptom of some health disorders, from distemper to worms. The old-fashioned name for distemper was 'the husk'. (See Worms and Distemper.)

But when the cough is a result purely of an irritation of the mucous membrane of the throat or the upper parts of the alimentary canal, or disorders of the lungs, then local internal and external treatment will give relief.

Treatment Make a strong infusion of liquorice root, using one tablespoon of the root or a one-ounce piece of the solid juice. Add one pint of cold water and bring to the boil. Add one teaspoon of honey to each tablespoon of the liquorice brew. Give two tablespoons before meals. Sage leaves, blackberry leaves, elder blossom, thyme, the whole plant – are good cough remedies, made in standard infusions. Sage is the best. Also blackcurrant jam, stirring one tablespoon of the jam into a cupful of water: add honey. Also a brew of borage or pine needles, a dessertspoon of each, finely cut, made as a standard brew and added to the liquorice.

Externally, friction the throat and chest with oil of eucalyptus, one teaspoon dissolved in one cup of warmed olive oil. Keep the area covered with heated towelling.

DENTITION (FAULTY) This is a modern development. Normal tooth quota is deficient, usually it is the premolar teeth, one or two missing, usually in the lower jaw. This causes a gap in the mouth, and food cannot be dealt with properly.

Treatment Man cannot give the dog artificial teeth! The only remedy is prevention through a natural diet of whole foods, and through selective breeding.

DIABETES This disease was a rare ailment of the dog until recent years, but it has now become quite a common one, in the same way that cancer has increased from rare to common. This incidence of canine diabetes is a severe warning against the folly of artificial diet; against the can of processed meat and the fancy carton of highly processed cereal known as 'dog biscuit'. Diabetes can also be caused by shock. There is also the insidious form of shock inflicted upon the sensitive canine body by repeated vaccinations of all kinds common to the modern dog. Veterinary analysis of blood and urine is necessary to detect diabetes.

Treatment   This requires a preliminary careful fasting, following the internal cleansing treatment, followed by the usual NR diet.

Avoid the use of insulin;   corrective diet is a far safer way of controlling and, in many cases, curing this disease. The cereal should be restricted, using rye in the NR diet, and this can be purchased from most grocery stores as a crisp bread. Use also as a cereal substitute carrots, either raw, grated, or lightly cooked. Carrots themselves, although often forbidden to diabetic cases, contain a natural-type insulin and are therefore really beneficial; so are Jerusalem artichokes. Medicines are powdered oak bark, a brew from shaved olive roots or from olive leaves, one teaspoon daily. Give also a daily dose of herbal antiseptic tablets.

DIARRHOEA   This is not usually a separate ailment, it is more often a symptom of some other internal disorder, such as gastritis, brought on by over-eating or through incorrect diet or the irritant properties of chemical preservatives present in most processed foods. Presence of masses of worms in the digestive tract, or as a symptom of distemper or other fever ailments, can cause diarrhoea. Correctly treated, diarrhoea is easy to cure and often proves beneficial to the later health of the dog as it can serve as Nature's method of removing a dangerous accumulation of toxic matter in the body. Therefore in herbal medicine, treatment of diarrhoea is opposite to orthodox. The latter aims at immediate checking of the bowel flow by use of starchy foods or blocking preparations of the kaolin class. Herbal treatment encourages bowel flow by the use of vegetable laxatives such as senna, and juices of figs and other laxative fruits.

Treatment All members of the onion-garlic family, also lemon juice, are specific remedies for diarrhoea, as they sweeten and soothe as well as disinfect the entire digestive tract. Fasting is essential in diarrhoea, for it is useless to burden the body with food of any kind at a time when all of the body energies are required for the removal of waste matter from the digestive tract. Food given at such times will merely ferment and further burden the sick animal. The fasting, apart from the giving of honey-lemon juice and herbal tablets containing garlic, should be maintained very strictly until all putrid odour and bad colour leave the bowel flow, then honey can be given both as food and healing agent. Apple juice is very healing in diarrhoea and can usually be given with benefit after the first forty-eight hours of the attack. (Now see the Internal Cleansing Diet, Chapter 6, for introducing milk and cereals, especially tree-barks' flour, which acts as an internal poultice, not blocking the digestive tract, but soothing inflamed areas with its vegetable jelly as well as nourishing the body. See also Dysentery, Chapter 3).

I have a typical report from Mrs J. Kennedy, of Evershot, Dorset, concerning a Pekinese puppy which had had intermittent diarrhoea for three *months* and had been on orthodox veterinary treatment throughout that time with no success. The herbal treatment and use of my tree-barks' gruel cured the puppy within one *week*, and there has been no return of the ailment. This same herbal cure has also won fame in the treatment of scouring sheep and lambs and has even cured many cases of the dreaded 'black scour' of sheep.

I recently used the gruel at the Dr Lytton-Bernard Ranch, Guadalajara, Mexico, on a wild raccoon cub, deprived of its mother and fading rapidly from scour. The raccoon grew into a healthy adult.

I again used the food with good success, when I was in charge of Professor Szekely's goats in Tecate, Mexico, for treatment of weakly kids and in hand-rearing kids. And while working on the third edition of my first canine herbal book I cured two orphaned hawks of chronic diarrhoea from which they were dying.

An effective treatment learnt in Greece is pounded sage made into small balls (honey can be used for binding the herb) and given as pills twice daily. An average dog would take a dessertspoon of the herb daily. Whin (blue) berries, also called bilberries, are another famous international cure.

DISTEMPER   Formerly I wrote a one-hundred-page book on the prevention and cure of canine distemper. This was included in its entirety in *The Complete Herbal Book for the Dog*.

Distemper in dogs is prevalent in most countries where the domestic dog is bred and dates back to the earliest centuries, and yet the cause of the disease has never been proved. Canine distemper is described in most veterinary medicine books as being a virulent, highly contagious ailment which is frequently accompanied by serious nervous complications. That is the orthodox description, resulting from unnatural treatments with sera, chemical drugs, and incorrect invalid diet. For my part, using simple herbal treatment, including fasting, I have found distemper easy to treat, speedy to cure, and devoid of any after complications. Testimonials world-wide, written in many languages, will uphold this statement.

That many breeders who have entire kennels wiped out by canine distemper, and many owners who have lost their pets over-frequently from distemper, are seeking the herbal treatment has been proved by the large sales of this herbal book in the countries in which it has been published: England, Australia, Switzerland, Germany, Holland, USA. In Switzerland it is veterinary surgeons who have translated my herbal books into Swiss-German.

The veterinary profession in most countries generally accepts nervous disorders as a usual accompaniment of distemper. And yet, out of the same thousand cases of this disease that I have treated, less than a dozen have developed nervous disorders, and in every one of those dogs the disease had been in a highly advanced stage before coming to me for treatment. I have never had a case develop either chorea or paralysis. What, then, can the reason be for nervous disorders being prevalent in one treatment and absent following a different one? I am convinced, and have proved countless times, that the main cause of nervous complications is the unnatural practice of giving food to invalid dogs when high fever is present, i.e. temperature around or above 103° F. During fever all the normal processes of digestion are suspended, all of the body forces being concentrated on fighting the bacteria which are causing the fever condition; food given at such a time poisons the entire system and seriously impairs the animal's power to conquer disease. In most cases the dog will put up a frantic struggle against the forced feeding, but occasionally, nervousness caused by the fever will induce a dog to eat up all food that is given to it. When, as frequently happens, forced feeding through the mouth proves impossible because of the dog's struggle against this, the hypodermic syringe is used, and such unnatural substances as brandy, salines, and even blood are injected into the animal's fevered body. If a dog does recover from such treatment, he is usually left permanently nervous, in poor condition, and very susceptible to skin diseases, the normal health balance of the body having been destroyed permanently.

Then there is the further unnatural treatment of serum

injections, the antibodies in the serum being supposed to aid the blood corpuscles in fighting the bacteria causing the disease. These shock injections into a disease-weakened body will often abate the cleansing processes of the case, and mucus discharges will cease abruptly; the temperature drops to normal and the animal is considered cured, whereas, in truth, the ailment has merely been suppressed, driven deeper within the body. After a week or so, it is common for the temperature of the serum-cured case to soar up again, and then invariably nervous disorders swiftly follow, with violent fits or paralysis. These symptoms are in turn suppressed by sedatives, and the dog then indeed passes beyond possibility of cure, and usually has to be destroyed. Nervous disorders (see Nervousness) can be cured by herbs, but they have proved difficult to cure when resulting from the unnatural treatment described above.

Symptoms of distemper are typical and easy to recognize. 'The husk', its old-fashioned name, alluded to the persistent, dry cough usually present in this disease. (Yet in some cases there is no cough at all.) Beads of pus form at the corners of the eyes and the eyes themselves are suffused with blood, especially the white, the inner lids being inflamed. The nose is hot and dry. As the disease progresses the eye discharge becomes copious and there is also similar discharge from the nostrils. The mouth smells fetid, the eyes turn very bloodshot, and often diarrhoea is present. The temperature next rises rapidly, and with this rise the dog becomes very listless and troubled and seeks a dark place in which to hide itself. Food is refused and there is often much shivering.

Treatment The dog must be fasted immediately (see Internal Cleansing Diet, Chapter 6). He must be isolated in a quiet, warm place, with a window sufficiently open to admit fresh air, day and night, oxygen being very important in this disease, or lung complications will develop. If the dog is being treated in a kennel, there should be a deep hay or straw bed provided and, again, ample fresh air. Herbal antiseptic tablets should be given night and morning, or simpler home-made pills from finely grated raw garlic, mixed with honey and a very little wheaten or other flour, to bind the mixture. The mouth and teeth should be cleansed morning and night, using very diluted lemon juice, one teaspoon of the pure juice (not synthetic) to two dessertspoons of water. It is advantageous if the dog also swallows some of this lemon water. Give several tablespoons each morning. Eyes and nose should be cleansed of mucus at least three times daily, using cotton swabs dipped into an infusion of any one, or a mixture, of the following herbs: rosemary, elder flowers, chickweed, speed-well, balm.

Any soreness of nostrils or eyes should be treated with an application of pure almond oil.

Honey-water should be given. If the dog will not take this, then give plain water and roll thick honey into small balls and push down the throat at what would have been meal times if the case were not fasting. Honey does not tax the digestion in any way; being predigested by the bees when in the hive, it is absorbed immediately into the bloodstream.

When the fever has ended, the dog can be immediately taken off the internal cleansing treatment, and the Natural Rearing Diet followed instead. During the treatment the dog should be taken outdoors sufficient times to relieve itself. The movement of limbs is beneficial, also the change of air.

If diarrhoea persists even after the fever has ended, add tree-barks' preparation to the milk. This flour will soothe the digestive tract as well as provide nutritious yet light food. Sprinkle a small half teaspoon of powdered cinnamon to every cupful of tree-barks' flour.

If all food is persistently refused by the dog even after

temperature has been normal for some time, a return of the fever can be expected soon, and the case must be fasted a further period until fever subsides.

Throughout distemper treatment, for at least three weeks or more, the dog's temperature should be taken night and morning. Use a clinical thermometer of the 'stub', not finely pointed, kind. The whole dietary regime of the case is dependent on the temperature readings (see p. 138).

Suggested times for honey, etc, are: 8 a.m., 12 noon, and 7 p.m. If the case seems exhausted, fresh grape juice or bottled or packet grape juice, the unpasteurized kind, can be given, or apple juice, fresh or bottled, can be given. Average dose of juice for a cocker-size dog would be two tablespoons, morning and night.

Distemper Complications   If the disease is treated in its early stages there will be no complications. Beyond the slight disability of a cough, discharging eyes and nose, bouts of diarrhoea, and some fever, the dog will keep well, and the disease will generally have run its course, and the case be cured, within three weeks.

In fact, it should be a general rule that any sign of 'off colour' in the dog, i.e. listlessness, lack of appetite, abnormal sleepiness, or shivering, should be treated immediately by fasting and generous use of antiseptic herbs, isolation from other dogs, and the taking of the case's temperature morning and night. If these precautions are always taken – and I have always taken them for my own dogs, goats, etc – there will be no distemper disease as we know it today, and certainly there will be no complications.

But if first symptoms have been neglected, or the case is very in-bred from weak stock, or has been vaccinated recently, then any of the following complications could occur, and some of them are severe and dangerous to life. These distemper complications are: nervous disorders, including chorea; fits; paralysis; meningitis; chronic diarrhoea; jaundice; pneumonia and pleurisy; bronchitis; deranged heart; ulcers of eyes and mouth; eye keratitis and more. (See treatments for all these ailments, in this chapter.)

Breeders' Reports on Distemper Cure

On account of the many new herbal treatments added to this new edition of my canine herbal, I now have space for only four reports, instead of the fifty reports published in the first English edition. But I think they will lead many dog owners to utilize my herbal work, for, as declared Mrs Joan Peck, of the famous Sakkara Salukis (whose salukis were cured of hard pad by herbal treatment): 'I have heard of many people being converted from the orthodox to the herbal treatments, but I have yet to hear of a single case of the opposite conversion.'

Report No. 1   Mrs Joyce K. Gold (K. J. Fryer), Oxshott Cockers, Rabley Heath, Welwyn, breeder of many of England's greatest cockers, and a famous judge.

For two years in succession I proved the complete success of your wonderful distemper treatment. Whereas in earlier years, puppies fed according to orthodox treatment when showing high temperature invariably had complications and generally died, following your treatment all my dogs made speedy recoveries and there have been no losses . . . I have told so many people what a safe distemper method this is, and incidentally have cured many different dogs by phone that way. I shall always bless the day ten years ago when I got in touch with you, for the peace of mind your treament of canine disorders has given me. I fear no illness now, as a few days' garlic treatment and fasting soon puts things right, but I must say my dogs keep *very* fit and free from ills, and it is many years since we have had anything serious to contend with.

Report No. 2 The Duchess of Laurino, Fenterwanson Pekinese, St Teath, Cornwall, a Pekinese authority.

I had twenty-seven Pekinese down with distemper, and treated them word for word as per your internal cleansing method. I lost one adult only. He started fits on the sixth day, but would have died whatever treatment he had been given, never having been normal. I had one young bitch which I despaired of saving. Her temperature continued for fourteen days. She was so weak that she could scarcely move, though in no way paralysed. Both eyes were badly ulcerated. Both lips and the nose sloughed off, leaving horrible pus on the open wounds. During all this time she had nothing beyond garlic and water. On the fifteenth morning I was rewarded by a wag of her tail. Next day she growled when I took her temperature; this was down to normal and remained there. I continued the fast a further five days, then commenced the milk-honey diet, and in one week she was out and about again, with no trace of weakness. The bare places around her eyes and mouth remained, of course, for some time, but in every other way she was a prefectly normal dog. She has since been shown several times, winning first prizes at championship shows.

The thing that impressed me most was that having shaken off the disease, even after prolonged fasts, there was no period of convalescence; they all seemed better in health than ever before. One dog contracted the disease despite the fact that he had been inoculated. Seven dogs who had never had it (given garlic), although in contact with the sick dogs, remained immune.

One bitch only has been left with any disfigurement, this

bitch continued running a slight temperature although apparently normal in every other way; unfortunately food was given, with the result that the temperature rose again and a second stage of the illness was entered upon with the tragic ending of an eye swollen almost entirely out of the socket and almost complete blindness in the other.

Before trying your natural method I have nursed dogs of various breeds with distemper, *only one of which I saved*. These I nursed by giving strong beef tea or chicken broth at two-hourly intervals, pouring it down their mouths when refused, also giving them beaten raw eggs in milk and occasionally brandy. The result seemed to be that the dogs' stomachs were always working overtime, also their bowels, and – as I have said before – they invariably died most painful deaths.

I find your treatment is a boon, as it is no trouble at all to carry out, and I am firmly convinced that if followed carefully and the dogs are kept clean and in warm, airy kennels, *all the dread of distemper can be forgotten*.

Report No. 3   Mrs Betty Butterworth, Rodworth Gundog and Cocker Kennels, Thonon-les-Bains, Haute-Savoie, France (now: Butterworth, 246 E. 53, New York, NY 10022, USA). Formerly Mme Coigny, Betty Butterworth was known throughout the French-speaking world, including North Africa, for her superb gundogs, which she exported all over the world.

When as Madame Coigny I ran the 'Of Rodworth' Cocker Spaniels, in Thonon, France, I started these kennels on orthodox lines, with cooked foods, and vaccines, and changed to Natural Rearing after three miserable years of endless work, dying dogs and worried perpetually by enormous bills for veterinary surgeons and chemists. I changed to Natural Rearing after a bad outbreak of hard pad in which I lost fourteen animals. The change was not easy, my faith not very strong, and the constant desire to return to the old method of drugs and inoculations was with me for many months. However, I persisted, as you know, and the results were beyond anything I had hoped.

During the next four years, with a basic stock of never less than twenty-five adults and rising at times to eighty dogs in the kennel, I lost only two animals and those through accidents and not illness. During these years, using only your method, I cured a newly purchased English bitch of hard pad. She was never isolated from the other stock and was the only case. Bored (if such a thing is possible) with the never-ending good health of my own stock and still not quite persuaded that the lack of illness was due to the treatment and feeding and not to my good luck, I began to search for sick dogs from other kennels and had among other cures great success in curing a bitch with bad chorea of the head and front legs, by fasting and then raw meat, seaweed powder, etc. She is now winning CACs in France for her owner and has bred some good stock.

We went through a local epidemic of hard pad which destroyed many dogs in Thonon-les-Bains, without one case in the kennels. And this, in spite of the fact that many of the farmers and sportsmen, having heard of the methods used in the kennels, would arrive with their dogs, bringing them on to the premises in all stages of the disease.

I think perhaps you realized my faith in Natural Rearing and my complete absence of fear when you brought your travel companion, Afghan hound, to me from Tunisia [Fuego – Turkuman Kakashah Larch-tree – later the sire of many US champions. It is now known that his ailment was the dread leishmaniosas, fly (midge type) borne, very prevalent in North Africa] with that strange skin infection from Arab desert dogs that we had neither of us seen before and which you so quickly cured with herbs gathered on our walks. It did not cross my mind to isolate your dog, or that any of mine would catch the complaint – none did, as you know. I had then and have now complete and utter faith in Natural Rearing, providing it is carried out thoroughly with no backsliding to drugs – plenty of free running exercise and good raw meat and strict attention paid to the usual kennel details of grooming and cleanliness. I attribute much of my success in the show ring to the health of the dogs, and I made champions of many of them, including Ch. Doebank Dominant of Rodworth, Ch. Walener of Ware, Ch. Silver Teal of Rodworth, Ch. Melforts Colleen's Joy. The black bitch that you admired, Rhapsody of Rodworth, is now owned by Baron de Boc and needs only her working certificate to become an International champion; and the blue roan puppy Rodworth His Majesty of Hearts, which you picked out, is already an American champion.

I hope one day to work again with animals and to enlarge my Natural Rearing experience with Farm Stock, but while I have had many opportunities to work along orthodox lines I confess I have not the courage to face again the disappointment, misery and death that are forever linked in my mind with the giving of drugs and inoculations.

Report No. 4 Viscountess Chelmsford, Beagles, etc, East Grinstead, Sussex. Famed as a judge of beagles, the late Viscount Chelmsford was one of the leading officials of the English Kennel Club.

By following your treatment, honey and water, fasting and using garlic, a litter of beagles, seriously ill, made a wonderful recovery from distemper; also one cocker bitch, which had been suffering from skin trouble for two years, made a rapid recovery. The treatment has given every satisfaction, and I am getting fine results. A Samoyed puppy had been digesting nothing before having the slippery-elm powder gruel, as prescribed; now all is perfectly digested, and she is making excellent progress.

[Later, Crufts 1953] Since using your herbal treatments in the early nineteen-thirties, I have had much time in which to fully test all that you advise. I am more convinced than ever before, and follow strictly the above advice in all your books.

See also my new book: *Three Virus Ailments of the Modern Dog* (Distemper, Parvovirus, Rabies).

DROPSY This condition of abnormal accumulation of fluid in the body is a serious ailment when found in the dog or cat. Herbal treatment has achieved numerous cures of dropsy, however, mainly because there are many herbs which are curative. These are: ground (dwarf) elder, dandelion, rosemary, parsley seed, sloe berries, yerba mansa (Mexican), couch grass. More rare, but proved excellent, are the reeds, Arundo donax (the great reed) and Arundo phragnitis (the bankside-reed). Macerate and give two teaspoons twice daily. The dog or cat should be fasted, given antiseptic herbal tablets and charcoal tablets. Follow the internal cleansing treatment carefully, but keep the case on a diet of fish (see Fish, pp. 20-1), in place of the raw meat, when full NR diet is resumed. Give internally quantities of any of the above-listed curative herbs. Give also buttermilk daily, as food or medicine. Give charcoal tablets.

DYSENTERY This is a very severe form of diarrhoea, which, if not treated properly and patiently, can have fatal results. There is often faulty temperature, either fever or subnormal temperature. Bowel discharge is very copious, very fluid, often orange in colour and foamy, with bad odour.

Treatment　Treat as for diarrhoea. Give chamomile tea, standard infusion, throughout: two tablespoons morning, midday, and night, average size dog. Apple juice, a tablespoon morning and night, should also be given. A good Spanish remedy for dysentery, which I have seen used in severe typhus disease, is rice water. This is both soothing and only mildly astringent without being binding. Take six tablespoons (level) of rice grains, one and a half pints of cold water. Bring to slow boil for two hours, keeping pan covered; remove from heat, and when tepid add two teaspoons honey and one half teaspoon powdered cinnamon. Give a small cup thrice daily, by spoon if necessary. Alternatively, give strong sage tea. Give also charcoal tablets and gruel. (See also Dysentery, Chapter 3.)

EARS: FOREIGN BODIES and WEAK MUSCLES　(For Ear Canker, see Canker)

Foreign Bodies　Often dogs, hunting around in country places, get thorny material or sharp grass spines in ears. Dissolve by dropping into the ear a saltspoon of oil in which rue or rosemary has been infused. Later dry out the ear with cotton swabs soaked in buttermilk or very diluted witch hazel. Continue twice daily until cured. Or infuse cloves in oil and use.

Weak Muscles　This condition is not really an ailment: it is more a question of show merit as to whether or not the ears of special prick-eared breeds stand upright or remain dropeared. But as herbs can help in restoring muscular tone, I have included this treatment.

Treatment　First, put the dog strictly on raw foods: NR diet, including uncooked (raw) maize flour in the cereal feed. This will stimulate general muscular development. Externally, using standard infusion, make a lotion of ivy leaves, but of double strength, i.e. two handfuls of ivy to approximately one half pint of water. When cool, add one teaspoon of witch hazel. Use the brew cold, massaging a small amount of it, twice daily, around the ear bases. Do not resort to taping or other artificial methods: rely on herbs and massage.

ECZEMA This is often Nature's method of ridding the body, especially the bloodstream, of accumulated toxins which have collected in the body from unnatural diet and/or lack of exercise. Also dirty, unbathed bodies are a cause. Streptococcal bacteria are often found in eczema pus, causing confusion with that disease. 'Strep' happens to be common bacteria found frequently where there is pus.

Treatment An infusion of nettle plant, or meadowsweet flowers, internally, with also herbal antiseptic tablets. In severe eczema a short course of internal cleansing may be necessary. Externally, apply a brew of bramble or elder leaves and flowers, or a mixture of both. Some can be given internally also.

EYE AILMENTS (See also Cataract, etc) The eyes are the health barometer of the entire body in man and animals. If the health of the body declines, the eyes at once also show decline and irregularities. I am convinced that the modern ailment of progressive retina atrophy is not hereditary but is caused by unnatural rearing through many generations until the eyes become completely starved of good healthy blood, are choked with impurities, internally and externally, and further afflicted by the air pollution of modern times and the use of poisonous chemical sprays on the home premises nearly every modern home has its spraying appliance for killing house flies, etc).

Cure must be internal as well as external: an immediate adoption of natural raw foods diet, remembering the essential daily provision of raw greens such as parsley, dill, celery, leaves, etc. Then substances known to be good for eye health should be included in the diet, such as grated raw carrot, sesame seed (tehena), honey, molasses, powdered carob pods, linseed in vegetable soup. For external bathing of sick eyes see Cataract and other eye ailments.

When foreign bodies get into the eyes, bathe with fresh milk. Also apply slices of raw onion to the eyes to make them run with eye fluids which will wash out the eyes of their own accord.

FATNESS   (See Obesity)

FITS   There are several forms of dog fits, caused by indigestion, or a distemper complication, or worms, or epilepsy. There are also the teething fits of puppyhood.

Treatment   Internal cleansing, with much use of honey. Give also grape juice, and black molasses. Herbs effective in curing fits are wood sage, poppy heads, skullcap, rue, hops and rosemary. Add minced raw lettuce and garden mint to the food, a heaped dessertspoon. For worm fits, see Worms. For epileptic, give strong doses of skullcap. An effective French peasant remedy is six mistletoe berries twice daily, before feeds.

Mrs G. Petter (of the firm of Petter Oil Engines, Yeovil, Somerset) sent me a dramatic report concerning fits cure:

I had taken my pet poodle to the veterinary surgery for destruction as his fits had been diagnosed as incurable. Returning from there I met Margaret Hemery [she now lives at Santa Inez, California and is well known in America as a judge of boxers and author of the book *Boxers* (Ernest

Benn)], breeder of Mayerling Boxers and Alsatians, who told me she had cured an Alsatian of 'brain' distemper by following your treatment, and to get back the poodle if it had not already been put to sleep. The dog was still alive. Mrs Hemery helped me and I carefully followed your treatment. The dog completely recovered and became very strong and normal.

Cures of fits with herbs have been numerous. Chances of recovery are greater when dogs have not been given any serum shots previously, or had suppression with 'quietener' drugs.

FLEAS, LICE, TICKS, AND OTHER SKIN VERMIN   These skin parasites are all blood-sucking and all do immense harm to the dogs which harbour them, especially to young stock; all dogs should be searched daily. The skin irritation caused by their presence keeps the dog in a constant state of unease, while the flea itself is known to be a cause of bubonic plague if carried by rats, and is also a carrier of a small species of tapeworm (*Dypylidum canicum*); the louse is suspect as a carrier – it is proved as a conveyor of typhus to humans – through its bite. The 'blue' lice or pigeon lice can cause a very painful skin condition of raw, inflamed patches, fever and discoloured teeth. Ticks can cause fevers in dogs, which can prove fatal.

Treatment   The first essential is to groom the dog and remove all loose hair, mats, scurf, etc. *Daily* brisk brushing and combing, morning and night, are very important in canine care. This friction of the hair and skin disturbs and harasses skin parasites, really troubles them and spoils their breeding cycle, helps evict and also kills some of them. A special fine-toothed flea comb is an advantage. Then bath thoroughly in a foamy bath of soap flakes, scrub well, also with a brush and using a bar of soap, preferably with olive oil. Do not forget to wash well the ears and tail. For perfect cleanliness, a second bathing with a good shampoo is advisable. External care is a first necessity. Precautions should be taken as to bedding. Do not use straw baskets or sacks, both of which provide excellent breeding places for skin parasites for such as fleas do not breed on animals but on the ground. Black specks seen on dog hair are dried fleas' blood, not eggs. The flea excretes this blood to feed the flea larvae on the ground. When the dog is fully dry, dust over the entire body with a herbal insect repellent, not forgetting inner ear flaps and under the tail. Avoid all chemicals: they are apt to do more damage to general health than the insects against which they are being used. A herbal rub for use when searching for vermin on the dog: moisten a pad of cotton wool or a piece of cotton cloth and sprinkle with a few drops each of oil of eucalyptus and spirit of camphor. This makes fleas easy to catch, and loosens lice and ticks. A clever gypsy tip for catching fleas is to moisten the human fingers with saliva. When the flea is touched, the saliva glues its leg mechanism and it cannot jump and escape. Saliva is also useful in removing ticks. In catching *lice*, search around on the floor at dusk, where the dog is lying. At that time lice are leaving the dog's body to degorge themselves of blood and can be picked up off the ground. The tiny ones can be crushed on the spot, or swept up in a paper soaked with paraffin, and burnt. In cases of severe lice infestation it is very helpful to spread sheets of white shelf paper beneath the dogs. The lice which drop off can then be clearly seen and killed.

Lemon Lotion   Save all used lemon halves and place them in a gallon container, at least twenty-four halves to one gallon. Place the jar or container in the hot sunlight or pour hot water over the lemon. Let the lemon remain permanently in the water until pieces begin to turn mouldy, then remove and replace with fresh ones, squeezing hard the old ones into the water. Do not throw away any of the old lemon water which then remains. Rub the lemon lotion well into all parts of the dog's body to expel skin vermin. A little may be dropped into the ears. For a stronger lotion, add the juice from two lemons to every quart. (Keep the jar covered with a paper top – not creased paper.)

Protective Lotion: against ticks and lice (not fleas which are too small and which should be killed on the dog by bathing, etc). I have made up a protective lotion which does cut down infestation by at least half. I aim at pungent smell and bitterness, which makes the dog's body *undesirable*. Into a pound-size jar, put two handfuls of herbal protection powder, preferably my formula, or powdered wormwood or southernwood; rue and St John's wort added improve the lotion, if available. Now fill up three-quarters with white beer and the rest of the jar with vodka. Cap well and place in sunlight (or in a warm oven, protecting the jar against breakage) to infuse. Shake well every day. After three weeks it should be ready for use. Do not strain, leave the herbs in the alcohol.

It must be stressed that it is useless to cleanse the dog's body of vermin while leaving his kennel untreated, for where there are but a few specks of dust a flea can remain and breed: and fleas, like most vermin, are extremely prolific. It is essential to the health of a dog that the kennel in which it lives should be lime-washed and rested frequently, also the kennel runs, which should be dug over and limed before being rested from use. No kennel or run ought to be occupied for longer than a six-months' stretch without a period of at least one month's resting. Wooden buildings and earth (or even concrete) runs provide a harbouring place not only for the external vermin, such as fleas and lice, but also for the eggs of

worms and for disease-provoking bacteria, which can remain
alive for many years in the ground, according to the finding
of Professor Antoine Bêchamp. Let it be known that real
infestation by skin vermin is not found where there are ideal
kennel and rearing conditions. A dog groomed daily and
possessing a tough skin – natural accompaniment of true
health – resists vermin. Cleanliness of animal and building i
the surest safeguard against vermin of all kinds, including
rats, mice, and cockroaches.

During the seasons of ticks and lice (and both these para
sites do have their special seasons worldwide – they are
generally most active at the time of high grass in midsummer
it is advisable to bring dogs indoors out of runs or gardens a
dusk. It is then that the parasites are most actively crawling
around looking for victims to suck their blood. If dogs canno
be taken in, then it is helpful to rub a few drops of spirit of
eucalyptus into their coats on top of the head, under the
brisket and above the paws on all four legs.

Flea Collars Avoid them. Any product which carries a warn
ing to 'keep out of reach of children' should be highly sus
pect. The dog expert, George Hampden Edwards, warn
against the dangers of flea collars. 'I would never use this laz
way of dealing with the flea problem, nor did we use the ora
method, the use of systemic drugs.' He states that the journa
New Scientist noted that studies by Walker and Stevenso
showed that where flea collars were worn, the animal's rec
blood corpuscle cholinesterase could drop to less than 20 pe
cent of pre-exposure. The chemical used on flea collars ha
been proved to be dangerous. This dichlorus chemical is also
used on house flies. I have found that the delicate tissues of
eyes and inner ears are damaged more than the fleas! I would
never use chemicals for my dogs. Collars of woven eucalyp
tus and other flea-repellent herbs – pennyroyal, fleabane

tansy – can be useful, especially if impregnated with euca-lyptus.

American veterinary doctor, Richard H. Pitcairn, in his excellent book *Complete Guide to Natural Health for Dogs and Cats* (Rodale Press), warns from personal experience against the use of flea collars. He states: 'They don't work. They are toxic. Some cats even hang themselves on them.' He also warns against flea 'tags' which are worn suspended from plain collars. He confirms that these appliances, which emit toxic gases (the flea-deterrent principle on which they work), affect not only the animals wearing them, but can also dam-age humans who may breathe the gas.

Herbalists, particularly in America, are supplying collars woven from herbs such as eucalyptus and pennyroyal, but although these are harmless they would have to be renewed frequently to be effective.

Herbs which fleas are also known to dislike are rosemary, santolina, chamomile, southernwood, wormwood and (strangely enough) celery and parsley tops when they have gone to seed.

My final advice is to powder the hairless parts of the dog's body where fleas most like to bite with a mixture of the anti-flea herbs listed, used in dried, finely powdered, form.

FLIES There is another blood-sucking skin parasite which attacks the dog in hot climates, though many dog owners remain completely unaware of its painful presence. Of the species horse-fly, but much more troublesome, this is a flat, yellow fly with big eyes. It flies on to dogs and hides itself in their hair and will remain there for days sucking blood if not detected. On long-haired dogs it is easily caught because it can be crushed into the hair. On short-coated dogs it is very difficult, as when attempts are made to catch it it leaps away to return later. When the fly is detected it should be crushed into a piece of vinegar-soaked cloth and killed. Note that it is difficult to kill. I call this evil insect the camel-fly, as it used to madden camels as well as dogs when I was in Tunisia. It is also prevalent in Israel during the summer months.

There is another species of fly which enters the nostrils of animals, especially sheep, but it can also infect dogs. It lays its eggs in the nasal passage. Remove by washing out the nostrils with Herbal Protection powder in water solution. Add several drops of eucalyptus oil to the lotion.

FUMIGATION Where there has been severe vermin infestation in kennels, there should be fumigation with either a sulphur candle or cayenne pepper. For either method, do as follows: first remove all dogs, then seal all doors, windows, cracks, etc, from the inside. Then light the sulphur candle and seal up the outer door also. If cayenne pepper is used, a paraffin stove should be placed in kennel or building, and lit; then on it place an empty tin. Pour into this one ounce or so of cayenne, and leave this to smoke slowly, sealing up the outer door also after exit. Allow the pepper to burn and smoke overnight in a completely sealed building. After fumigation with either sulphur or cayenne pepper, the place should be well ventilated for at least twenty-four hours before dogs are allowed to enter it.

The advantage of the old-fashioned wooden-tub kennel or old packing case was that, being cheap, it could easily be replaced by a clean, new one, burning up the old and all worn ova and insect vermin along with it! Expensive kennel buildings are a mistake. Better to have many cheap ones *which can be rested and/or replaced sometimes*.

In warm weather all bedding should be removed. Clean sacks can be given if desired.

A Herbal Insecticide lotion During wet weather it is not possible o use a dry, powdered insecticide. Here is a home-made otion of proved effective action and entirely beneficial to anine health. Pour ½lb herbal insect repellent powder, such s my own formula – five-herbs powder which I call Herbal 'rotection powder – or powdered derris root or tobacco dust, nto a glass flask big enough to hold two quarts (the big ottles sold with spring or purified water are suitable). Next, dd two ounces of oil of eucalyptus and one quart of pure lcohol (or white beer can be used with excellent results). Cork tightly to prevent the escape of the natural herbal oils eleased by the alcohol. Set this to steep for four days. Shake he contents well, morning and night. The lotion must now e filtered to prevent over-fermentation. Do this through a rge funnel packed with cheesecloth or cotton. Have ready nother large bottle capable of holding at least two gallons, or ave two bottles capable of holding one gallon each. The lcohol lotion can now be diluted to a quantity of two gallons nd yet retain pungency sufficient to destroy skin parasites. If ere is any fermentation later on, it does not matter, it will ncrease the pungency of the lotion, and it is for external use, ot internal.

If the odour of eucalyptus oil is objected to for house pets, en the more expensive oil of rosemary can be used, the ame two-ounce amount. Good herbal stores stock this or can btain it on order. For use, rub the lotion well into the skin ver the entire animal, but keep from close contact with the yes.

ASTRITIS AND GASTROENTERITIS The former comes from ulty diet or worm infestation; in the former cause the ouble is especially due to the long-term feeding of cooked ods and to the giving of irritant appetite-stimulating drugs a 'condition'-powder form.

Treatment (See Diarrhoea) An infusion of parsley leaves i
also recommended. A long fast is often necessary. When the
fast has been ended, use should be made of steamed parsle
roots, well minced and fed with the cereal. (No salt is to b
added during the steaming which should be carried out in th
smallest possible amount of water, that water being retaine
and mixed in with the cereal – a dog can obtain all the sa
necessary to health through the medium of the seawee
powder, as given in the NR diet.) In orthodox treatment it i
usual to limit drinking water strictly. In contrast I give as muc
fluid (chamomile tea) as desired.

GLANDS (Swollen in necks, colds, distemper; see also Mil
Glands). The treatment for dropsy is exactly suitable for glan
dular disorders, including swelling (see Dropsy). Externall
apply hot lotion made by dissolving powdered seaweed in hc
apple cider, or hot oil of camphor can be used.

HARD PAD AND BRAIN DISTEMPER (CANINE ENCEPHALITIS
The disease is usually classed as a virus ailment and, lik
distemper, its real cause has not been proved. I link the diseas
very closely with canine distemper, and I further believe fror
careful observation that it is an actual form of distemper. It ca
be cured by the same method, though it is usually held to b
nearly incurable by those who treat the disease by orthodo
methods. I consider the disease curable, though not so easil
as distemper, for animals which produce hard pad diseas
symptoms have reached a very substandard state of healtl
and their bodies will require very careful and prolonged inte
nal cleansing and dieting in order to attain normal health. It i
far more prevalent in Europe than in the Americas. Commo
symptoms are: diarrhoea, which is seldom absent as an earl
symptom of canine encephalitis; also an excessively moi
nose, usually with drops of water continually appearing ther

similar moisture is frequently found around the eyes, although there is no yellow mucus discharge, or from the nostrils, typical of common distemper. There is always a raised temperature, for there cannot be inflammation of the nerves without any indication of fever, and it is the general body nerves which are first inflamed – one of the causes of diarrhoea, for diarrhoea can well be produced by purely nervous irritation of the intestinal tract, and therefore nothing at all is gained by merely checking the diarrhoea flow and leaving the nerves still sick and irritated. There is always a staring coat, and usually the inner earflaps are very hot, and some discharge is also seen there. It is always much later, and sometimes not at all, that the foot pads – and in some cases the nostril pads – thicken and become leathery, and finally harden and become almost without feeling, in the same way as skin areas do after long-lasting follicular mange – only in hard pad it is more exaggerated. With this stage are found the brain symptoms, shown by the staggering gait of the affected animal and constant whimpering which cannot be suppressed by command, the dog acting involuntarily, and desribed as 'insane', until in the last stages it is a raving madness similar to pure meningitis.

Internal Treatment Similar to canine distemper, although more intensive, for hard pad is indeed dangerous, whereas distemper is a simple disease to treat. Once the typical symptoms have been verified – diarrhoea, very wet nose (and possibly eyes), fever (usually a temperature of an unvarying 103° F) – the only possible treatment to prevent death is a complete fast on honey and water only; or herbal teas and honey, such herbs as sage, thyme, marjoram. Add a sprig of antiseptic southernwood to the tea herbs, if available. It should be grown in every garden. (Try to obtain pure honey, not the syrupy, often pasteurized substitute for the pure thing.)

Medicine should be: a daily dose of antiseptic herbs, especially garlic and rue, double the dose as prescribed for canine distemper, given each morning. Follow this with a twice-daily dose of a brew made from potato peelings as follows: shred a small cupful of potato peelings; pour over this three cupfuls of cold water; bring to the boil and simmer for about ten to fifteen minutes, until the water turns light brown. Allow the peelings to stand and steep off the fire for at least two hours, then squeeze out the juice. Dosage is two tablespoons twice daily for big breeds; one tablespoon twice daily, medium breeds; two teaspoons, small breeds. Give also a large dose of vegetable tablets, made to my formula, and being pure chlorophyll extracted from nettles and meadow grasses and comfrey. A laxative is necessary during fasting – see Internal Cleansing, pp. 145-8). This appears to be a large amount of dosing, but the disease is a serious one, and it is far preferable to have such work in the early stage of the disease, and cure resulting, than the enormous amount of work entailed in caring for a case of brain fever, which state, when allied to hard pads and nostrils, becomes very serious indeed.

If there are definite brain-disorder symptoms, skullcap treatment should replace the potato brew internally until the nerves are soothed and normalized.

Hard pad taken before brain disorder sets in is curable. I have achieved many cures with the fasting-herbs-potato treatment. (Potato-skins' brew has a remarkable effect on diseased tissue, and combined with garlic, on my prescribing, has even cured the considered-to-be-incurable fistulous withers of horses. This treatment was given much publicity in agricultural journals in England, aroused wide interest and helped to achieve my BBC radio talk on many kinds of animals which I have saved with herbs.) Peasant farmers in Ireland use potato skins for sick animals and, incidentally, were using bread mould (penicillin) dissolved in water – as animal medicine and also for their own ailments – long before English scientists ever 'discovered' the medicinal value of the mould fungi group.

It is interesting to note that in an old herbal book of the Mexican army, a brew of potato peelings, used externally, is given as a cure for the dread typhus fever.

External Treatment Make poultice boots from a piece of cotton, linen, or sacking – nothing woollen – spread with a plaster of pulped, boiled potato peelings, or oatmeal or barley flour. The boots must be kept in place with adhesive tape or some strong tape. Change the boots every day, allowing half a day *without* boots before each new application. The boots must be very loose-fitting around the pads, but tied firmly up the leg.

Warning The cessation of the diarrhoea is no sign of a full cure; normal temperature, maintained steaily for three days, is the most favourable sign of cure, and permits milk and, later, other foods to be added to the honey-water diet. Continue to take the temperature daily; in case of relapse, continue for at least eighteen days in all hard pad cases.

A further warning is against the use of any drugs of the sulphonamide group. The indiscriminate use of these *highly dangerous* drugs is quite possibly one cause of this disease, allied with the presence of toxins of the distemper type. It is notable that in cows – animals which react very badly to chemical medicine – sulphonamide treatment is frequently followed by disease of the hoofs. There may well be some link between the modern popularity of these dangerous drugs and the corresponding frequency of hard pad and brain distemper, for mental disorders are another common after-effect of the sulphonamides.

Prevention of hard pad As I have already stated, Natural Rearing is a sure preventive. When dogs are known to have been exposed to infection, disinfect their bloodstream with Nature's most potent disinfectant – herbs, especially garlic and rue. Be unfailing in this habit.

Finally, I want to bring attention once more to the prevalent error of classifying all sorts of minor canine disorders as being hard pad, now that this disease has 'leapt into popularity', taking the interest from the once equally important streptococcal infection disease. The late Leo Wilson, FZS, wrote sensibly on this matter:

> In assessing these cases [hard pad], however, one must always be sure that diagnosis has been correct. When a 'new' disease becomes an epidemic the label is applied loosely to a variety of cases which may not be the disease at all and consequently the cures effected do not help in the fight against the major foe.

The spreading of superstitious fears concerning diseases of humans and animals is often the work of serum 'merchants' preliminary to their marketing of a new serum.

I am grateful to Miss May Rodgers for her dedicated report on her success with hard pad treatment, which I give herewith. Miss Rodgers writes with authority, having cured the disease on three occasions. Leo Watkins introduced her work as follows, in a paragraph headed 'Hard Pad Cures' in his London Wire (*Our Dogs*):

> More than one of my readers mentions the use of garlic in one form or another, both as a cure and preventative. One writer, Miss M. Rodgers, of Leeds, is particularly warm in her praise of garlic, which she used in conjunction with starvation treatment. She claims successes against Hard Pad with this method as long as twelve years ago.

'Miss May Rodgers, Gledhow Chows, 66 Upland Grove, Leeds, Yorkshire.

'I first had this disease in my kennels about twelve years ago, and treated the dogs as for distemper. I wrote to Juliette de Baïracli-Levy (when she had distemper kennels in London, at Talbot Road, Bayswater) and she wrote back that she had never come across the disease where the pads hardened, but would like to know the detailed symptoms, and what progress I made, etc. I kept her fully informed, and she said she thought that, seeing one particular dog was ravenously hungry *and* running a temperature, his brain *must* be affected (which proved to be). I eventually got him better, but he was always nervous. His litter brother (my blue stud Chin-Cha – retired from stud now) would not have *any* food, not even honey or milk, and he had no after-effects.

'Since this experience I have had Hard Pad twice in my kennels, the last time four years ago, when I again wrote J. de Baïracli Levy, and she suggested that I poultice the feet. Though I do not poultice any more, my experience having found foot coverings to be unsatisfactory.

'As to *treatment*: (I have not so far lost *one* dog or bitch.) I starve the same as for distemper (internal cleansing), and give garlic night and morning – one tablet per dose. I do not touch the dog's pads except to rinse them with aired boiled water once or twice, *until* the dog starts to tear them off himself, then I leave them *severely* alone. Rinse the mouth and clean the teeth with lemon and water (one and a half teaspoonfuls of pure lemon juice to two tablespoons of water) and do not 'fuss' the dog, simply keep him quiet and warm (not in a hot room, he does better in his own kennel). I have found that the cases want plenty of water and also that the temperature is often *below* normal at commencement, though it rises as the dog's feet harden.

When the foot pads are coming off, I put my dogs on the milk or milk-and-water diet, with addition of a teaspoon of honey. The slippery elm, etc., powder form, is good to use before the dogs are returned to normal diet, especially useful to check the tendency to bowel looseness which is also one of the true early symptoms of Hard Pad disease (the only other commencing symptom that I have observed is the dog's habit of walking very *carefully*, as if he had a touch of rheumatism in his front legs. There are no other symptoms at commencement).

'I hope that my experience with Hard Pad will be of use to other dog owners. I shall be very pleased if I can help to cure this disease and encourage other people to try this simple treatment.'

Mrs Gisela Meyer-Frank, Karl-Muller-Str, 8, Dusseldorf, Germany, tells me how herbal method is becoming accepted in her country. She cured her own Afghan of a severe attack of hard pad, using my herbal treatment under supervision of her veterinary surgeon who was 'very interested in your method. We read together some brand-new veterinary books and I found the same as you told me: garlic, green herbs, raw food, eucalyptus, and watercress, against Hard Pad.'

HEART WEAKNESS AND DISEASE (See also Worms, Heart-worm) The treatment of all the many types of heart weakness and disease is similar. In the main, the heart should be relieved of all unnecessary work, through diet reform to reduce superfluous flesh and free the bloodstream of toxic accumulations which are so damaging to the heart and the bloodstream in general – for the health of the heart is largely governed by the state of health of the entire blood system of the organism. Exercise should not be curtailed. Active exercise is necessary for complete food digestion; otherwise, the bloodstream becomes impure and the heart is further harmed.

Treatment The specific remedies for heart disorders are: rosemary and honey. An infusion of rosemary should be used, one level teaspoon of pure honey being added to every tablespoon of the rosemary infusion. Rosemary herb has all of the three medicinal properties necessary in heart treatment: it is tonic, cleansing, and also a nervine. Honey is the only known heart stimulant and restorant which is not a drug and which is not habit forming. Dandelion leaves and watercress should be given daily on the meat feed, for their rich iron content, and the potassium and copper content of dandelion which has an important effect on heart restoration. Regular fasting and use of mild laxatives, such as rhubarb root or senna, should also play an important part in all heart treatments.

Avoid digitalis, the popular heart medicine; from the simple herb foxglove the chemists have made a dangerous medicine. Flowers of lily of the valley are a very good heart tonic, but expensive. Heartsease (wild pansy, *Viola tricolor*) is another well-proved heart tonic and remedy. It is very good against heart 'stress' in all racing creatures, horses, greyhounds, pigeons. To make a syrup of heartsease, start with a strong brew of the herb, one tablespoon to a half pint water, add a half teaspoon ginger powder. When tepid, strain, add a half tablespoon honey and golden syrup.

HEAT RASH AND HEAT SPOTS   The dog in the wild was a cave dweller. To this day he likes to lie in cool and shady places and suffers during hot weather if cool places are not available. I've noted that in very hot climates the dog sleeps by day and becomes active by night. During very hot spells, red blotches or spots may develop all over the dog's body.

Treatment   Give barley and sour milk in the diet, both being active blood coolers. Give a mild laxative such as rhubarb-dandelion pills at night. Do not give any fats in the diet. Externally: by day apply raw cucumber juice or lotion of elder blossom or meadowsweet. Some of these herbs can also be given internally further to cool the blood. By night, powder with fine oatmeal or talcum powder, preferably from a spray.

HEPATITIS (*Liver Disease*) This disease has a short incubation period and can develop and be passed on to another dog within three days or so. There is often some pus in the eyes, bad breath, great lassitude, rapid wasting, irregular bowel action. This is one more hitherto rare disease now considered as common. That it is so severe and so general, and attacks an organ greatly influenced by diet, is one more proof of the terrible harm done to dogs by unnatural diet.

Treatment Isolate the case owing to its contagion. Treat as for jaundice (see Jaundice). Keep the case quiet and warm, as temperature often drops below normal.

HERNIA (*especially umbilical*) Hernias in the dog and cat are usually umbilical. In the cat this may be congenital whereas in the dog it is usually caused by rough treatment from the dam at the time of birth. Umbilical hernia is when, under the skin but through the navel, a portion of the intestine protrudes. A prominent hernia in a young pup may have gone away as the stomach area muscled up and hardened. In any case, even if the hernia continued into adulthood I would not approve treatment by surgery because internal harm may be done.

Treatment I learnt of an amazingly simple treatment from a vet in Greece for curing umbilical hernias in young pups. The affected pup is merely put on to its back, then the human thumb is brought down with hard pressure on the hernia, which will go back into place like a press-stud. This will very often effect a permanent cure in as little as a minute. Failing this, apply a mixture of the astringent, witch hazel extract, one dessertspoon, plus one dessertspoon well-crushed ivy leaves (common tree or wall-climbing ivy, of course, not poison ivy) and one dessertspoon castor oil. Mix well together and massage into the area morning and night for five minutes, for many weeks until cure is achieved. If this is unsuccessful, then I consider it better for the dog to live with the hernia than to risk surgical treatment.

Finally, prevention should be mentioned. Do not let the mother treat her whelps roughly at birth. She may fling them about in her nervous excitement, especially at a first birthing. Therefore stay with the bitch throughout her whelping and prevent her from treating the pups roughly and thus causing umbilical hernia. Calm down the dam, and remove the puppies from her into a box padded with warm flannel cloth and placed by the mother's side, returning the pups to her when the entire whelping is over.

HIP DYSPLASIA This abnormality is shown by a stumbling gait of hind legs. Faulty diet, deficient in natural bone-forming foods and lack of exercise are the basic causes. It is well known that puppies are not born with hip dysplasia, though there is a tendency to inheritance if the parents have not been well reared. The abnormality develops slowly over the years when insufficient dietary care and good exercise are given to keep the limbs normally healthy.

In a normal hip, the strong ball head of the leg fits perfectly into the socket hollow and is held there by healthy tissue and ligaments. In the abnormal hip, the ball head of the leg is frail and slips around in the hip socket instead of fitting perfectly. This loose fit puts a heavy strain on the ligaments and tissues of that area, and in time severe lameness develops and the affected dog moves in pain. The ball end can also crumble a little.

Treatment There is none. As with every canine ailment, the most successful and sure deterrent is *prevention*, which means following strictly a Natural Rearing diet plus provision of ample exercise. Give bone-forming cereals, especially oats, sufficient fibre, and natural calcium in the form of big, raw bones to gnaw, raw eggs, but not too many eggs – three or four a week for three weeks in the month would be ample. Give also buttermilk, cheese whey, white cheese – they are all calcium rich – grated coconut and sufficient safe oils (sesame, sunflower, corn). I evolved a special meal for growing pups and juniors (though adults appreciate it too and I enjoy it!). It is specially to grow strong bone and, in addition to home-milled (by windmill) whole-grain cereals, not toasted, it contains such extras as carob flour, malt flour, ground liquorice and beneficial herbal spices. Dog owners can make their own.

Natural vitamins, particularly C and E, should be given, for they are known to prevent bone weakness. Many firms in the USA now specialize in natural vitamins and in England there are Larkhall Laboratories, Charlbury, Oxford. Dried fruits are all potassium rich, especially figs and dates. Give crushed sunflower seeds, also drops of evening primrose in milk. Evening primrose grows wild on sand dunes or can be obtained from herbal shops.

Once the disease has developed, feeding raw, finely minced comfrey leaves or giving comfrey tablets has achieved cures. Because this disability is difficult to mend once the bones have deteriorated, aim to avoid its development. Dosage of comfrey would be one tablespoon minced comfrey leaves with midday and evening meal, or three comfrey tablets morning and night for an average dog, to be given five days a week until ailment is cured. Honey may also be given. It is very bone building: it says so in the Bible.

HYSTERIA The causes are many, the disease certainly not being caused by any specific bacteria, although many canine writers still claim that that is so. The many causes can readily be summed up in the two words which occur with such frequency in this book – incorrect rearing. Three contributory causes are: the presence of worms in large numbers, hereditary nerve weakness, and – boredom. The third cause, that of boredom, deserves further comment. The unnatural imprisoning of dogs in kennels for long intervals, or in small runs, without the provision of sufficient daily outside exercising, leads to a form of either mental depression or unnatural excitability in dogs so treated, a dog's nature being such that it is supplied with very highly developed feelings of affection and also the faculty to take a keen and intelligent interest in the life of its own home – or kennel. Therefore, as is often the case, the dogs are cut off from all outside interests, and the kennel owners have little time to spend in the company of the dogs, which are kept more as mere breeding machines than living creatures. It is understandable that the dogs so treated should become fretful and also ultra-sensitive to the slightest degree of excitement, and therefore prone to develop attacks of nervous hysteria at the most trifling cause. If this hysteria is to be prevented, it will therefore be seen that two reforms in the common life of the kennel dog are necessary: correct feeding, in order to ensure strong nerves and at the same time prevent worm infestation, and the provision for the dog of a way of life in which it can fulfil those special purposes for which it was created, namely, that of being friend, champion and guard to man, and also destroyer of harmful rodent vermin and serpents. Then, above all, supply ample, active exercise.

Treatment When a dog develops attacks of hysteria, the most important contribution towards successful cure is rest in a darkened room, combined with fasting, the full internal cleansing treatment then being followed, with a return to a fluid diet whenever further attacks of the hysteria occur. The same herbal treatment as for fits should be followed. I must also mention the fact that because hysteria is such a noisy and generally alarming ailment, breeders are frequently over-anxious to keep the dog artificially quiet by drugging, the commonest medicines used for drugging being bromide and luminol. These two drugs have been wittily and truly described by a medical writer as being 'those super Shylocks which demand a thousand per cent interest for any temporary relief they give'. How true indeed that statement is! The prolonged use of bromides (and other 'doping' drugs of that class) develops a peculiar state in the body. There is the case of the bromide drugs (the medical term for that state is bromism), a few symptoms of which state are herewith given: dilated pupils; development of acne on various parts of the body, especially the head and face; a fetid, bromine breath; slow and feeble action of the heart; breathlessness; cold extremities; various mental conditions, such as weakness and confusion of mind, and a type of general intoxication.

The one medicine that can be safely given in hysteria is the skullcap infusion: that herb is no suppressive drug, it actually feeds and builds the nerves as well as soothing them. Rose-mary, rue, hops, lime blossom, lemon verbena, vervain are also good. The one food which has a curative effect in hysteria is honey. Rose-hip syrup and blackcurrant syrup are beneficial; dissolve field poppy flowers or poppy seed heads in them.

INGROWING EYELIDS This is often hereditary and can be cured only by surgical operation. I have found the trouble frequent among wire, smooth, and Airedale terriers, and many breeds of toy dog, especially poodles. The operation is simple and inexpensive. Bathe the sore eyes with rosemary infusion, this being antiseptic and healing. The following herbs all make good eye lotions: balm, chickweed, dock, quince, seeds, poppy heads. Diet can also greatly improve eye health. Linseed soup, finely grated raw carrot, cooked carrot, watercress, molasses and all whole-grain cereals.

INTERDIGITAL CYSTS   (See Abscess)

JAUNDICE   This ailment is commonly called the 'yellows', named for the yellow hue that dyes the entire body surface, even the gums and eyeballs. The causes of jaundice are many, and include: congestion of the liver – frequently brought about as a sequela of distemper, or through a severe chilling; blocking of the bile duct by the passing of a gallstone or the entrance of a round worm. There is also a form of contagious leptospiral jaundice said to be caused by rats, typical cases, however, of this having been found where no rats or mice could possibly have been responsible; serum injections are given for this jaundice. They are given with the admission of 'kill or cure'; they usually kill. There is also preventative inoculation, which itself is more deadly to young stock in its after-effects than are even distemper inoculations. The one unfailing jaundice preventative is sound rearing according to the laws of Nature.

Treatment   Infusion of dandelion leaves and root, the two infusions to be given mixed together in equal parts; for preparation of the root, see preparation of couch grass (under Bladder Troubles), also toad-flax or blue pimpernel in infusion. An infusion of rhubarb stems is also very effective: two ounces of stem to one half pint of water cooked into a thick syrup, with honey added. And pomegranate juice when in season, an average dose being two dessertspoons morning and night, or St John's wort. Externally, a paste of common mustard can be made into a poultice and applied hot to the region of the liver. A course of internal cleansing, with garlic dosing, must be followed; but when the milk-honey stage is reached, the milk should be given sour and skimmed, and only half the usual quantity of honey given – both measures being intended to relieve the work of the liver, which is the organ of the body most concerned in fats and sugar digestion and storage. Therefore strictly limit intake of fats of any kind. Make use also of the 'bitters' in herbs especially blue gentian, the root, finely grated, a half teaspoon twice daily, centaury, whole herb, as a brew, and wormwood and southernwood, in powder form, as pills.

Extraordinarily good results have been obtained in the treatment of jaundice by the above method, despite the fact that jaundice is considered one of the most fatal of all canine ailments.

Note I must repeat that the entire success of the jaundice treatment depends upon strict fasting long enough for the liver to have become cleansed, and the bile to have been cleared from the bloodstream and body tissues. Several weeks of dieting on NR gruel, which is so internally soothing, can save life in severe cases, plus use of the curative jaundice herbs already listed, especially blue pimpernel infusion, one teaspoon of herb to every two tablespoons water.

KERATITIS This is a clouding over of the eyes; their natural clearness vanishes and they often turn an unsightly solid-looking blue.

Treatment Give the dog a period of internal cleansing. Give as medicine: carrot juice, carrots – shredded raw and/or cooked, corn meal, linseed tea, to improve the health of the eyes through diet.

For eye-bathing lotion, see Cataract treatment.

KIDNEY TROUBLE, INFLAMMATION, ETC (See Bladder Troubles for complete treatment.) An infusion of parsley leaves should replace the couch-grass infusion. The internal cleansing method has given outstanding results in kidney diseases; numerous incurables have been cured. Cleavers plant infused in cold milk is effective. Also parsnips, grated, raw, can be rolled into balls, with thick honey. Also recommended, the 'silk' of corn. (See Corn, p. 26).

Shrunken Kidney and Pulpy Kidney These are two modern ailments which strike particularly at the young. It should be remembered that the kidneys are a major internal cleansing organ of the body and that they have to handle all the impurities which get into the urinary system as well as having to cope with the impure water which is now quite general worldwide instead of the former sparkling water from clean springs, streams and wells. The kidneys cannot cope with the strain imposed on them and abnormalities develop, from inflammation to actual shrinking and wasting, or turning pulpy, as does that other tender organ, the liver, when diseased.

Treat all kidney derangements as advised for bladder troubles, and remember the soothing and healing bacteria- and disease-fighting properties of pure honey, further improved by blending with barley water, and that Nature provides many herbs for cure of kidney troubles.

LEATHER-SKIN (OR ELEPHANT SKIN) DISEASE The cause of this serious ailment may be abnormal secretions of the glands; in one form it is the pituitary gland, in another it is the sebaceous glands: sometimes a hormone deficiency. Origin is considered to be internal as with most skin ailments; even ringworm and mange are influenced by internal health. In leather-skin, the skin thickens like leather; if not checked and if the condition spreads unduly, there will be no recovery.

Treatment   Treat as a glandular disease (see Obesity). Give an abundance of seaweed and garlic internally; externally massage the skin with garlic infusion in castor oil (see preparation under Abscess).

LEPTOSPIROSIS (*Leptospira canicola, Leptospira icterohaemorrhagiae*)   We can classify these two ailments as 'new'. Almost unheard of when I commenced veterinary work nearly fifty years ago, they are now so commonplace that dog owners, especially in Europe, are being urged to have their dogs vaccinated with a triple vaccine, to protect not only against canine distemper and hard pad but also against these two forms of leptospirosis (and while going 'the whole hog' in vaccines, why not a fourth shot to protect against contagious hepatitis?). It is good to know that one of the world's most famous dogs, Ch. Shirkhan of Grandeur, of America, has never been vaccinated against anything, and yet he has travelled with his owner, following his great triumph of Best of All Breeds, at Westminster Show, New York, 1959, attending championship shows throughout the United States and winning Group after Group prizes, and has also travelled on invitation to Venezuela.

Healthy dogs do not get leptospiral infections; they, again, come to the ones reared by unnatural methods. *Leptospira canicola* is often called 'the lamp-post disease', as city dogs, especially males, are said to infect themselves from sniffing around urine-soaked lamp posts, on which infected dogs have urinated. The bacterium is corkscrew-shaped and infects the kidneys. Infected dogs become very emaciated, blood is often passed in the urine. As many as 50 per cent of dogs in most cities of the world are said to be infected. One should count NR dogs among the disease-free other 50 per cent because they will not get the infection. Healthy kidneys resulting from healthy feeding give them their immunity.

Symptoms of *L. canicola* are: refusal of food, vomiting, fetid breath, abdomen tender to the touch, blood sometimes passed in the strong-smelling urine, and a rapid loss of weight.

L. icterohaemorrhagiae is supposed to be rat borne and affects the liver, causing internal bleeding and rapid death. A normally healthy liver will resist attack. I should also say that leptospiral ailments are often made scapegoats for common canine distemper. Cases which have been vaccinated against distemper cannot be admitted by the veterinary surgeon as having developed the disease, therefore it is called leptospirosis instead: little wonder that the percentage of town dogs suffering from this 'new' disease is now put as high as fifty dogs out of every hundred.

Treatment Exactly as for canine distemper. Fasting and resting the case, giving antiseptic herbs, also honey. For the kidney infection, see also Bladder Troubles; for the liver infection, see Jaundice.

Although leptospiral jaundice is considered to be almost invariably fatal, many complete cures have been achieved using simple herbal methods.

LIMBS, BROKEN AND FRACTURED Damages to limbs are quite frequent in the dog; it is usually the long bones of the leg which are injured, occasionally the ribs. There are three kinds of fracture: simple, when the bone is broken in one place only and there is no wound; compound, when there is a wound in addition to the fracture and communicating with the fracture; and comminuted, when the bone is smashed in several pieces.

Treatment The simple break does not usually present much difficulty; it is with the two other forms that much care has to be used. The first thing to do is reduce the injury – which means the setting of the broken bones in their natural position. The next thing is the splinting and the bandaging of the injured parts, securing the limb in such a way that the broken bone ends are prevented from moving out of place once they have been set, keeping the bones in rightful position in order to ensure the uniting of the broken bone-ends: this process is always a difficult one owing to the dog's natural dislike of any coverings on any part of the body, especially on the legs. (It is known that when wild deer sustain a broken leg, as the result usually of a fall from a cliffside or elsewhere, they keep the injured limb inactive and raised from the ground, until the breakage has healed. Such breakages, through falls, are not uncommon among wild deer, whose dread of man as a result of the terrible hound-hunting persecution to which they are subjected causes them to inhabit dangerous cliffsides and other similar places. But I have yet to see a wild deer with a crooked leg.) I think that it might often prove the best policy where a nervous dog is concerned to allow the dog to heal its own limb, merely keeping the dog confined in some quiet place until the limb has healed sufficiently to allow the taking of active exercise again. Internally, give an infusion of broom, the tender shoots and the leaves of that shrub having remarkable power in promoting the uniting of the ends of fractured bones. Wild animals with broken limbs will seek out the broom bushes at such times. Give comfrey, a common wild herb, also cultivated as cattle fodder, and another very important bone-healing herb. Indeed, a common name for comfrey is 'knit-bone'. Give this herb internally, chopped finely and mixed with the food, also as an infusion, standard method, two tablespoons dose, morning and night. Then further use the infusion on cotton cloths, cold, thoroughly soaking the cloths and padding them around the broken limb: if a plaster setting is used, this is not possible. As the cloths dry, more brew should be added, to make a cold herbal pack. Comfrey encourages the speedy formation of new bone. A substance, allantoin, is largely responsible for comfrey's bone-knitting property. I have seen amazing results in bone healing from the use of comfrey. One case was a saluki male puppy at Yodfat farm in Israel. Both hind legs were broken below the stifle, the result of an attack on the puppy by a wolfdog. Comfrey was used, both internally and externally, and within a month both legs had mended and the pup could run normally.

Drinking raw goat's milk, in the experience of a famous goat breeder, Mrs Lucy Tyler, Flemington, New Jersey, is a great aid in mending broken bones.

When I was in Texas, USA, recently, I met Miss Mac-Donald White, of Associated Press, a follower of NR for years. She brought me a black and tan Afghan hound to see. The Afghan had fractured a foreleg some months before. I was asked to examine her legs, as the owner vowed I could never tell which one had been broken. She was correct, I could not tell, even when in movement. The Afghan had been treated by the herbal method that I am here describing.

But when the fracture is of such a nature that the bones must be kept in position by splinting, then the greatest care is required to make sure that the splinting does not interfere with the blood circulation, which interference would naturally prevent all healing and could produce a septic or even gangrenous condition. It is this very factor which makes me opposed to the modern veterinary method of tight setting in plaster of Paris, or other settings of that class. Such a setting might answer for a simple fracture, but in a compound or especially in a comminuted fracture, plaster of Paris settings are not to be recommended, and I have formed this opinion from bitter experience. I have seen the badly fractured leg of an exceptionally healthy hound puppy set in plaster, the hair having been clipped off the leg and the plaster applied to the skin without any padding of any sort to relieve pressure, the result of such unnatural treatment being that so much fluid and bad blood collected in the pinched limb that at length the swollen leg burst its way through the plaster, the condition of the limb then being such that destruction of the puppy was necessary.

I most definitely prefer the old-fashioned method of splinting and lightly bandaging, for that method does at least allow the leg to breathe – and when the bandaging is lightly applied, does certainly permit normal circulation, which, of course, is essential to healing. There is a gypsy method of setting broken limbs – which is still in use on sheep farms in the West of England – and that is setting in 'containers' made from plant stems or tree branches. When a dog, sheep, or other animal fractures a limb, either a stout cabbage stump or elder branch is taken, and the pith removed from the centre, the stalk or branch then padded with some soft material (sphagnum moss, because of its antiseptic properties, would be excellent for this, or the healing elder leaves), and the stalk or branch then fixed round the fractured limb, and held in position by light bandaging. If the limb is a very broad one, then several stalks or branches can be placed edge to edge and then lightly bound in position. The advantages of this natural herbal splint are many: both stem and branch are porous and admit air to the limb; they are slightly pliant; their inner sides are soft and will not form hard ridges in the manner of plaster; but, above all, the herbal splints are themselves possessed with healing properties, and will therefore encourage Nature in her natural reparative work. For instance, the old herbalists used to prescribe cabbage water as a lotion for bathing bruised, swollen, aching, or gouty legs. The leaves of the holly tree, when trimmed of their prickles and bruised, and applied to fractured limbs in the area of the fracture, are claimed by the gypsies to have remarkable powers of uniting the bone ends so that they are left in as strong a condition as they ever were before the fracturing.

Holly should also be given internally, as a standard brew, one tablespoon of leaves to half a pint of water with honey added. Give one tablespoon dose three times daily. Another important advantage of herbal splints is that if the injured limb should swell it is only necessary to loosen the bandage and increase the space between the splint edges encircling the limbs; whereas, in plaster settings, it would be necessary to strip off the plaster altogether for resetting, which would certainly cause the animal much pain and at the same time might well cause a further breakage of the injured bone ends.

The main points of natural treatment of fracture are, therefore: a natural setting of the limb, which means very light splinting and bandaging at first, during the time that the injured limb usually is swollen and tender (the splinting can always be tightened as the leg heals and the swelling disappears); the most careful daily inspection of the limb to make sure that the circulation is not being interfered with (not possible when plaster settings are being used); the provision of both quiet and rest, the dog not being permitted to take any active exercise at all for the first ten to fourteen days following the fracture of the limb, and, further, a course of internal cleansing to help the body in its healing work; fasting and fluid diet, followed by only very light diet – of importance when no exercise is being taken. *Also important*: take the temperature daily. A rise in temperature is a warning of complications and the limb must then be examined for over-tight bandages (or plaster), etc. In fever, fast the case.

When ribs are fractured, the area of the ribs should merely be wrapped around with a broad bandage placed so that the broken rib ends are kept in position but not made of a tightness to interfere with the animal's breathing. Rest and dieting are the other essentials. Bind bruised holly leaves, trimmed of prickles, over the rib area, beneath outer bandage, to increase healing.

Further observations on broken limbs: Modern treatment for broken bones is to be condemned: it is unnatural, expensive and trouble making. X-rays are in general use and are in themselves very dangerous. I have noticed that, when X-rays are taken, human patients have protective covering against the rays, but animals have no protection at all. Sterility can be caused by X-rays of hind limbs. I am also against the modern use of metal plates, screwed into broken bones to hold them. They can cause permanent trouble, so refuse them.

LIVER AILMENTS   (See Jaundice and Hepatitis)

MANGE   This is a severe parasitical disease which occurs in two forms, sarcoptic and follicular, the former being the more common of the two and the more contagious, but fortunately the more readily curable. As mange attacks also the fox and wolf, there is indication that it can be equally parasitical upon the quite healthy animal; therefore, keep stock away from other animals showing signs of mange skin disease.

The two kinds of mange parasite are small, louse-type mites, invisible to the naked eye. They bury beneath the skin and increase with great rapidity. Cases of follicular mange often look as if they have been sprayed all over with gunshot, so numerous are the skin eruptions. The skin also turns elephant grey, hair falls, and an unpleasant mousy smell becomes noticeable.

Sarcoptic mange is often confused with eczema and vice versa. But there are differences. Eczema means the formation of small mattery sores, spotty eruptions, while mange usually shows large wet patches and especially favours the back and back of the neck. There is also a falling out of the hair in mange, whereas in eczema the hair usually becomes matted with pus, but remains on the body. The presence of other skin vermin, especially lice, will also set up skin irritation which can be confused with mange or eczema; the smallness of the common dog lice makes them difficult to detect.

Treatment This, understandably, should be external principally, but in order to effect a complete cure, the state of the dog's general health should be improved also, for the tough, vital skin of the dog in sound health offers much resistance to the mange parasites: it is usually the skin of sickly animals that is attacked. Some animal experts go so far as to say that mange can be cured entirely by corrective dieting and internal medicament. I consider that patient external treatment also is essential once the teeming parasites have established themselves in the skin tissues.

Complete fumigation of collars, leads, grooming equipment, kennels and runs is essentail (see Fleas, etc).

Herewith are four effective cures for both forms of mange. All are non-chemical and do not contain grease, which I consider to be very detrimental in the treatment of parasitical skin ailments, for it protects the tiny parasites and they feed on it.

Bath the dog thoroughly before applying any of these following treatments, using both soap flakes and a bar of olive-oil soap or coconut shampoo. Repeat the bath once each week throughout the treatment.

Herbal alcohol lotion (See Fleas for recipe)   The lotion must be applied to every inch of the dog's body, not forgetting the very tail tip and around the toes; only avoid the eyes and genitals. Friction well into the skin.

Lemon peel lotion (See Fleas)   When pomegranates are available, their peel can be added to this lemon lotion with great advantage to the treatment. Use the skins from three pomegranates to every nine lemons.

In sunless localities the lemon skins must be treated with hot water and simmered for several minutes, keeping the pan covered. Then remove from the flame and allow to steep. Do not take the lemon peel out of the water throughout its use. Its powers will be improved by adding some Herbal Protection powder of bitter herbs.

Garlic lotion   Follow the recipe for herbal insecticide in alcohol, as given under Fleas, but add finely minced garlic, six whole roots (approximately forty small cloves), to the herbal powder, using the garlic in place of the oil of eucalyptus.

Wormwood, violet and red clover lotion   Take a handful of each of these herbs: for the wormwood, the whole herb; violet, the leaves; clover, the whole plant. Pour over the herbs one quart of cold water, bring to a boil, and simmer for approximately three minutes. Keep covered throughout. Steep and use. Do not strain.

Garlic-elder lotion   Slice up three whole roots of garlic, consisting of about twenty cloves, and add to this two handfuls of finely cut elder leaves and stalks. Place all in a pan with one quart of cold water, bring to a boil, and simmer slowly for half an hour. Keep covered throughout. Remove from heat. Do not strain. Allow to brew for at least seven hours, still keeping covered. The lotion is then ready for use. Soak large pieces of cotton or towelling in the brew and friction the entire body very well. Two to three tablespoons of the brew can also be given internally early morning and at night.

For further internal treatment, if the case is very badly infected, a short fast may be necessary to clean the bloodstream. Give strong doses (double normal dose) of herbal antiseptic tablets – Herbal Compound.

Before closing this section mention should be made of constitutional hereditary mange, found especially in chows and dachshunds. Animals infected in this way should never be bred from. Unfortunately this rule is often ignored if a dog possesses good show points. Treatment for such mange is largely *internal*. Make much use of seaweed, giving a double dose, also herbal antiseptic tablets. Feed a strictly NR raw foods diet.

Mange cure from Helen Balk-Roesch, Loerrach 2, Baden, Germany:

I owe you a debt of gratitude in connection with your herbal canine book. I raised my small Scottish terrier according to your method. Friends of mine, the Gerhard Gunthers, also of Loerrach, brought me their year-old dog of the same breed. He was suffering from follicular mange and the attending veterinary had already decreed the killing of the little dog, as well as the complete disinfection of the apartment.

I bought your herbal book of which I had heard. After ten months of constant devoted care, I was able to return the dog to his owners, completely cured. Nobody would have believed it, but with the use of garlic inside and out, complete recovery. The illness was incredible. Not one hair

on his whole body, sores full of pus and with deep holes so
that one could see almost to his bones in many places. It was
a difficult task, but well worth it. Now Bimbo has a beautiful
coat like my own two Scottish terriers, which I bring up
exactly to your diet chart. *My Nature dogs differ markedly from
other dogs, not only in their behaviour and intelligence, but also in
the thickness of their beautiful coats.*

Another triumph was the whippet bitch, Laguna Lady
Lightfoot, owned by Mrs Leah Gut, of Wangen bei Olten,
Switzerland. This bitch, bred in England, developed severe
follicular mange. Veterinary college examination and diagnosis decided 'Hereditary follicular mange, at least one year
arsenic treatment, cure unlikely, not to be bred from.' My
treatment was followed, using bitter herbs powder in alcohol;
the mange was cured in a month and she later was highly
placed in shows. One judge, Bill Siggers, found her 'in excellent condition'. She also won challenge certificates in Italy and
Switzerland and whelped litters from which came many champion whippets. Not one of her pups developed any mange.

A right-up-to-date follicular mange cure: a Shar Pei, 'Khan'
owned by Linda Rupniak of Northampton, England, showed
no response to orthodox treatment – his skin was pitted with
holes, his condition serious – but was totally cured on my
herbal treatment so that he was able to qualify for Crufts and
has become a big winner. It is notable that when mange is
cured, not by suppression of symptoms but by internal cleansing of the body, the case passes on to its offspring its acquired
immunity to this serious ailment.

MENINGITIS   (See Hard Pad)

METRITIS   Metritis is a disease of the womb, which affects
bitches of all ages, including maiden bitches, and is more

common than is generally supposed; many bitches suffering from vaginal discharge are undiagnosed cases of metritis. The cause of metritis is usually held to be a germ which attacks the womb, but I have more faith in the less-known theory: that metritis is nothing more than a symptom of severe catarrh. The word 'catarrh' is derived from the Greek and means 'a flowing down', and this flow of mucus can well occur in any part of the body where there are mucous membranes; we thus get colitis in the bowels, metritis in the womb, and so forth. The disease is distinguishable by an unpleasant-smelling discharge flowing from the vagina, the discharge being of a pinkish hue, and when very copious is usually accompanied by a rise of temperature.

Treatment An infusion of wild rose fruits (or garden rose). When not available the leaves can be used, but they are far inferior to the fruits – the hips. The hips should be well crushed, and then brewed in the usual way. Strain well. The infusion is improved by the addition of witch hazel extract, one half teaspoon of the witch hazel to each tablespoon of the infusion (average dose). Douching with an infusion of lavender flowers and leaves is also helpful. In severe cases the lavender infusion can also be given internally, at midday, in addition to the morning and evening dose of rose-hip infusion. The other part of the treatment is fasting and internal cleansing, making good use of the internal disinfecting, and mucus-expellent, powers of antiseptic herbs.

Mention should be made of the herbal cure of the Dandie Dinmont terrier, Ch. Peachems Wannie Blossom, owned by Mr and Mrs E. Stubbs, of Angmering, Sussex, the terrier being such a famous one. Three veterinary surgeons had seen this case and no hope of cure was given; a slight promise of recovery was given *only* if the bitch were operated on for the removal of the entire reproductive system. With herbs and the bitch's own good health powers from her careful and Natural Rearing, she made a full recovery without operation.

This letter reached me in 1984 from Sue Collyer, Nagazumi Afghans, Oak Tree Cottage, Bunkers Hill, Ash, Sevenoaks, Kent:

> I have tried to use your NR method as far as possible since I read your Herbal for the Dog over ten years ago and found results very satisfactory, and none of my Afghans or my Bichin Frise is vaccinated. I used your methods especially well four years ago. One of my Afghans, six weeks in whelp, was running free in a field with friends' dogs. One collided with Zuki, the bitch in whelp, knocking her badly. Next day she was very ill with a nasty-smelling discharge and fever metritis.
>
> She then showed all the signs of being in labour and about to miscarry. She was passing disintegrated pups. A vet I consulted wanted to carry out a hysterectomy as he believed the womb was infected from dead puppies. I took her home, refusing such an operation. I would rather let her die than be so mutilated.
>
> Following your book's advice, I fasted her for five days and dosed her with Herbal Compound tablets and an infusion of rose hips and witch hazel, plus raspberry leaf birthaid tablets which my bitches always receive. All my neighbours collected rose hips for me! The discharge was cured, all fever went and Zuki seemed recovered. Then about ten days later I felt the movement of a puppy yet alive! She carried six pups to full term, whelped easily in one and a half hours (she was seven years old by the way) and I kept a beautiful domino colour from that litter. Zuki has gone from strength to strength since – and her pups have won well at shows.

n his book, *Old English Sheepdogs in Australia*, George Hampden Edwards describes how he saved an OE sheepdog and her litter from metritis, using my herbal method.

MILK GLANDS TROUBLE 'False' milk is often troublesome in pitches, also excess milk, following weaning. The former is generally met with in maiden bitches who produce milk at the times when, if mated, they would have been having a litter; however, brood bitches also can develop this 'false' milk when they have not been mated. The treatment for this trouble is exactly the same as for metritis (which see), but with no external douching, and the treatment naturally being used in a much shorter form; for example, one day's fasting, followed by two or three days' milk-honey fluid diet. In this ailment it is more beneficial to use the milk in a sour state: in that way it becomes somewhat laxative; honey should still be given. The external treatment, in this trouble, is the bathing and massaging of the hot and inflamed milk glands with an infusion of mint leaves (common garden mint) or mint and lettuce leaves. An excellent alternative treatment is external bathing with dock and elder leaves. With this latter treatment I have had great success in curing mastitis in cows and goats. Internally, give twice daily in doses of two tablespoons a brew of wood-sage or common sage.

The same treatment should be followed for cases of excess milk in the dam following the removal of her weaned puppies. It is the over-early removal of a litter which is frequently the cause of the dam's excess milk, early sales often being the motive. The unnatural over-early weaning of puppies is one of the greatest causes of poor health among dogs; a well-bred brood bitch will be able to feed her litter until the puppies reach the age of seven to eight weeks, and longer, the puppy weaning not commencing before the fourth week, when fresh goat or cow milk can be given, soon followed by tree-barks' flour, raw meat not being introduced into the diet until the fifth week.

MYXOMATOSIS This terrible plague disease of rabbits so far has not harmed many dogs, even those which have eaten diseased rabbits. The best safeguard against all disease is healthful diet and internal disinfecting with garlic, etc. If such disease should develop, treatment would be on hard pad lines. (See Hard Pad.)

NERVOUSNESS This is most frequently a hereditary or psychological ailment, best cured by careful breeding-out through strong-nerved stock, and patient, intelligent hand ling of the nervous case. I, personally, have restored many a nervous animal to becoming a well-balanced, normal one - dog and horse. Diet and herbs can, however, also play a helpful part.

Treatment Short cleansing fasts. Use of leaf-plasma tablets (a great natural nerve tonic, very rich in iron and iodine); sea weed, raisins, egg yolks, molasses, bran, honey, nettles (used as a 'soup' for soaking of cereal biscuit meal), wheat germ flakes or oil. In cases of true nerve sickness, skullcap rue, rosemary, vervain, peony root, valerian, lime blossom hops, field poppy, are all very helpful, given as a standard brew. Give seaweed too.

OBESITY This condition is generally more prevalent in bit ches than in dogs, and is frequently of a glandular-sexual nature. Advanced obesity can be very serious, and is not only a certain cause of barrenness in bitches, but also a cause of premature death. An abnormal accumulation of fatty tissue is not merely a harbourer of toxic accumulations, but also puts great pressure on the blood system which has to pump its way through the semi-diseased (fatty) areas of the body. Great muscular development is very different from flabby fat, and when the condition of an animal is being judged in the show ring, due merit should be given to muscular development and there should be penalization of fatness. Most dogs are shown far too fat because judges seem to prefer this; a dog by nature and natural conformation is a lean creature, active and speedy of foot.

A corrective and very laxative diet is the main method for the internal breaking down of fatty tissue, the diet to be interspaced with short fasts of from two to three days on a diet of water only, with a daily senna laxative dose, of approximately two or three senna pods for an average size dog. This will clear away fatty substances dissolved during treatment. External improvement must be largely regulated by abundant exercise, the exercise becoming increasingly strenuous as body improvement takes place. Encourage swimming in river or sea.

Castration of male and spaying of female animals, because this interferes with normal rhythm of the body and normal glandular health, creates obesity of a cruel and often unsightly form, and shortens life.

Treatment A daily dose of an infusion of rosemary herb. The daily use of parsley and dandelion on the meat feed, together with daily dose of seaweed powder, because of its tonic effect on the glandular system. Starchy foods should be greatly restricted, and to every half pound of whole-grain cereal used, one handful of raw bran should be added. Feed finely grated raw cabbage and onion mixed into the food and let raw and cooked carrots replace at least a quarter of the starchy cereal ration. Bitches and stud dogs should be allowed to lead normal sex lives, for lack of this is the commonest cause of the prevalent fatness seen among pet dogs and bitches.

PANCREAS (*over active*) Once rare in dogs, now quite common. Normal food digestion is curtailed and there is rapid loss of weight.

Treatment As for Jaundice, although not allied. Put the case on a very light diet avoiding all fatty foods. For herbal remedies give pills of minced gentian root (see Parvovirus), also give charcoal tablets and pills of goldenseed herb. Fresh-pressed grape juice will also refresh and cleanse the pancreas.

PARALYSIS This is not necessarily a distemper sequela, paralysis, especially of the hindquarters, often attacking young and aged dogs. The trouble is caused by pressure on the roots of the nerves in a limb, or a group of muscles, or pressure on, or other interference with, the brain or the spinal cord itself; in the case of paralysis of the hindquarters, constipation may be the cause; a serious blow or fall can also bring on paralysis – car accidents are a typical cause; it also can result from severe worm infestation. Paralysis of the hindquarters is a fairly common hereditary ailment of the dachshund and Pekinese breeds. But excellent results have been obtained with herbal treatment. Indeed, hundreds of cases, many of them condemned as incurable, have been restored to full normal health.

Treatment (See Chorea and Distemper) The skullcap infusion should be replaced by one of sage leaves. Give also grape juice. Externally, an infusion of mustard seed, one teaspoon of seed to one cup of boiling water, should be massaged twice daily into the paralysed areas. Mustard powder can be used in place of seed, same quantities; merely dissolve in boiling water and apply rather hot. Give cayenne pepper tablets to stimulate the blood: two tablets morning and night is the average dose.

In my many cases of veterinary work my most spectacular

cure was with a case of paralysis – a pedigree Swaledale ewe with total paralysis of the hind legs of three months' duration. The ewe had become paralysed during the Great Snow of 1947; being especially valuable, she had been kept alive to await my expected visit to the farm – Kitley Farm, Arkengarthdale, Yorkshire. The limbs were cold and lifeless and covered with 'bed' sores. The exact canine paralysis treatment as given here was prescribed. In ten days of treatment the ewe was standing; in three weeks she was running so swiftly that she could no longer be caught for administering her medical treatment. The paralysis has never returned and the ewe has since given birth to one of the best lambs in the flock. In Arkengarthdale she is known as 'the miracle ewe'.

There comes to me from the same district, Swaledale, one of those 'dramatic' veterinary reports which make my herbal work seem worth while, and I am therefore persuaded to include the cure here in the text, as it is concerned with paralysis. From Mrs Gladys Hutchinson, Helaugh, Richmond, North Yorkshire:

I know you will be pleased to hear that a policeman all the way from Yarm brought a black Labrador bitch for me to treat by your method and thereby save, for the vets said that no more could be done for her. The police at Reeth told him to bring the bitch here, where your herbal methods are used. It had paralysis of the back legs. I did all that your treatment said, and in a *week* had the Labrador walking and going out rabbiting with my husband, in fact I could not believe it myself. The policeman said he was going to take it straight to the vets to show them the dog that would have had a grave if it had not been for herbal treatment. He wishes to thank you.

PARVOVIRUS (CPV) Parvovirus means 'The Little Virus' (*parvo*, small). It would require a booklet to describe fully this so-called 'new' canine ailment which has claimed its millions of victims worldwide, to say nothing of the countless more deaths unrecorded because the owners of such dogs did not know what had killed their animals. Parvovirus has only been around since 1980, it is believed, and it has gone in waves, both in the numbers of recorded cases, from high to low, and in the severity of the disease itself, from very strong to rather mild.

Strong or mild, however, experienced veterinarians describe CPV as the 'most horrible, terrifying and dangerous' of all known canine ailments and as being a true killer. From what I have seen I can agree about the 'horrible' quality, but not so much with its described dangerousness, because I believe that a dog raised well, according to the strict laws of Nature as to diet and exercise (and the, let us say, only mildly polluted environment) *can* resist CPV and the others of the ever-growing list of canine virus ailments: all of them.

When my own Turkuman Afghan hounds caught up with this ailment in Greece, they provided me with ample proof, but more important is the worldwide testimony in support. From the thousands of dog owners and breeders who follow Natural Rearing methods, there comes conclusive proof of the immunity of healthy animals. In fact, not one has reported to me a single loss from CPV, yet countless have had direct contact with CPV cases which died immediately afterwards.

Although it may seem unbelievable, it is true, as those who work with herbal products on my behalf can testify; unbelievable to me because I know that some people who claim to follow Natural Rearing do so in only a limited way (failing particularly in the provision of ample exercise and of truly clean earth in kennels). A last-minute change to a previous edition was initiated by Mrs Helen Cramer of Oyster Bay, New South Wales, Australia, collie expert and judge, who wrote, 'There is still plenty of parvovirus around in Australia, but the true Natural Rearing people have had no problems from this ailment.'

Living isolated as I do on a Greek island, I had not had personal contact with CPV until travels in England and on the Greek mainland in recent years, especially in the early 1980s, the peak years of the CPV epidemic. I received reports, however, typical of which was this from Sue Collyer, Nagazumi Afghans, Ash, Sevenoaks, Kent, and concerns not only the CPV ailment itself but the failure of attempted vaccination protection. She reported numerous failures and of the policy of many breeders to vaccinate only their more valuable show-going dogs, because of the high cost of the vaccine, and to leave unvaccinated the less valuable dogs. In many cases the vaccinated dogs took CPV and died and the others, despite the fact that they had been in close contact with the affected dogs, never developed the ailment at all. Her own Afghan hounds, many of them very young, had been at shows, standing next to dogs which died from CPV days afterwards, but had not developed the disease.

There has been much written concerning the development of sterility for both dogs and bitches as a result of CPV vaccinations or of orthodox treatment by drugs after the development of the disease.

My views on CPV agree with those of Douglas B. Oliff, Wyaston Bullmastiffs, Wollaston, Lydney, Forest of Dean, Glos, who feels that it is probably a mutation form of canine distemper virus, which in turn gave place to a far worse virus ailment, hard pad, and which in turn has spiralled more dangerously into CPV. What next? Douglas Oliff, who is a writer about the bullmastiff breed, is an international judge and has followed my Natural Rearing for his hounds for nearly forty years, fully shares my opposition to unhealthy and unnatural vaccinations of any kind. He has noted the adverse effects of the various vaccinations in relation to normal fertility of dogs and CPV vaccine seems to be worst of all in this respect, paralleled only by a vaccine against a parasite, heartworm, which has caused widespread sterility following its use. My latest news from Douglas Oliff, who is always very up to date in the canine scene, is that not only is there widespread concern among breeders about sterility caused by vaccination, but also concern about subsequent health decline.

In a very recent letter to me, the cocker spaniel expert, Kay Baldwin, Vailotest Cockers, 256 Willesden Lane, London NW2 5RE, shares remarkably closely Douglas Oliff's view I have long noticed that it is from the experienced breeders that one gets really important findings. She writes:

Do you have any opinion on the shrunken kidney disease which has stricken so many young cockers? I feel strongly that by inoculating against kidney and liver infections, plus distemper and hard pad and now parvovirus, at such a tender age and generation after generation, that something permanent has happened to the chemistry of our canine friends and that Nature is taking her toll for all the poisonous substances which have been introduced into such tiny bodies. I remember well that we managed to nurse distemper in the old days before the first distemper vaccine came along.

I feel that having found a 'stop' to distemper, Nature came along with hard pad – and so the next inoculation was added. In the course of time Nature has come through with parvovirus, and now they are groping in the dark – using vaccines about which they are unsure of the time they will give immunity and having very odd and unpleasant side effects (from what I hear).

Distemper, after all, was only an intense cleansing effort of the body and, when sensibly treated by fasting and use of cleansing herbs, was quite beneficial, never dangerous unless interfered with by attempted quick suppression of the symptoms.

A recent article by Kay White in *Dog World* (UK), was entitled 'We must change our ways to combat Parvovirus'. She wrote:

> Veterinary surgeons from all parts of Britain gathered to discuss their worries about CPV and vaccination regimes, and it was evident that they were very worried indeed. One vet described CPV as 'this terrifying new disease' . . . Distemper virus is fragile, easily killed by frost or sunshine, or an average standard of cleaning. *Canine Parvovirus is different.* Parvovirus persists against all but the most rigorous cleaning of walls, floors and ceilings; it may still come into a kennel or home on inanimate objects which have brushed against a dog's coat or on shoes or tyres, etc. There is a tremendous amount of Parvovirus around everywhere in the environment, and a special concentration wherever dogs congregate . . . The important thing to remember is that no vaccine can offer *total* protection and breeders must take other precautions.

Symptoms, cardiac type There are two types of CPV and I shall begin with the type that always affects the heart and is the quickest killer. This type is almost exclusive to young pups and occurs immediately after weaning when the disease-protective properties present in maternal milk of all animals, including humans (thus the vital importance of breast feeding), and known as antibodies, begin to weaken and fade. The general danger time for the cardiac type of CPV is from six to nine weeks, and is proved to be parallel with the weaning time of the litter.

Cardiac form of CPV is very distressing and usually fatal: no wonder that experienced veterinary surgeons describe this disease as terrifying. The affected pups huddle away from the light, breathe painfully, and suffer internal cramps as the heart muscles are attacked by the virus. The limbs collapse and often even the neck muscles cannot support the weight of the head, which then hangs painfully. Death comes speedily to the totally collapsed puppies, and the mother, if a witness, is greatly distressed. If the mother is young she may go down with the ailment herself, but more likely it will be the form of CPV which attacks more adult dogs which will end her life later.

This other type, which is equally prevalent but is less deadly, takes the form of very acute gastroenteritis. It shares one likeness that is typical of and almost exclusive to (except for rabies) the cardiac form and that is its very speedy development and contagion. The CPV virus can manifest itself within only hours of the time of contact with an infected case.

Both forms can be airborne, or carried from inanimate articles which have merely had contact with the body of an infected dog, or can be carried on human clothing and shoes. To sum up: dangerously contagious, both forms.

Symptoms, gastroenteritis type These are a very distressing and almost uncontrollable vomiting, which brings on deep exhaustion. This form of vomiting often brings on bleeding from mouth and bowels as internal blood-vessels are ruptured. Yet other CPV cases do not manifest internal bleeding but have a much stronger type of diarrhoea which has a very putrid smell.

In all cases a morbid interest in water, as in rabies, is typical. The cases sit by their water dish, but seem reluctant, afraid, to drink. Further, also as in rabies, there is a profound change in the eyes, which not only sink rapidly into the bone sockets, they have a changed expression – squinting, glazed and non-focusing.

Another typical symptom of this type of CPV is very rapid dehydration, an all-over shrinkage of body flesh so that the coat hangs loosely, the eyes become cavernous and the tail droops. Within a day or less a formerly fat puppy or young adult begins to look like a skeleton.

Yet another typical symptom of CPV, and this time a compensatory one, is the rapidity of recovery once the case has resisted the virus through its own attacking antibodies. Those cases on the road to recovery will be seen to repose themselves into sleep in a dark corner, fast from food and water, and in as little time as overnight or a mere day, show recovery. Desire for water and food returns, the faeces harden and lose their bad odour, and the mouth smells clean.

Fever may or may not be present in this gastric form of CPV, but, if present, it is generally high, over 104° F is typical.

Treatment This must be *immediate* if one is to save parvovirus cases: immediate, as in cases of poisoning. Simply treat as for poison, with the exception of the poison forms which attack the nervous system and require sedation as well as internal cleansing. But let me start with the longer-term curative treatment which – now that we are aware of the presence of this new canine virus ailment and know also of its killing rapidity – necessitates planned preventive vigilance.

The dam of the litter-to-be should be the first stage of CPV prevention. From the day of mating she should be dieted carefully, getting only the best of natural foods to ensure the development of puppies of maximum health. She should also be given much daily exercise, an essential in pregnancy. The next stage, when she is nursing her litter, needs equal care: she should be fed an abundant diet of natural feeds to give great health, in turn, to the pups she is nursing. Harmful early weaning should be avoided (see puppy rearing, p. 86) and she should be fed protective herbs against both worm ova and virus ailments which may be passed through her milk flow (see care of the brood bitch, pp. 72-5).

A healthy bitch can nurse her litter as long as sixteen weeks. This has been quite typical for my Afghan mothers and for nursing bitches of many other breeds when on Natural Rearing, particularly those which have remained more 'natural' and less domesticated, such as salukis, golden retrievers, Rhodesian ridgebacks, etc. Bitches are helped, and nursing strain lessened, if pups are given shallow dishes of water to drink, from two weeks of age, when their eyes have opened.

Health-giving puppy diet of raw foods is the next barrier against CPV, and general day-by-day good puppy care to ensure all-round strength and natural resistance to all types of disease.

The actual treatment is as with Poisoning (which see): fasting, of course, and giving urgently very strong laxatives to sweep out the virus. Senna pods and castor oil are given and dosage of both is extra large. In the case of senna, whereas three pods would be sufficient for an average size dog, seven pods should now be given: soak for seven hours in one teaspoon of cold water per pod with a pinch of powdered ginger added. Remove the pods and add some honey to the liquid to induce the dog to take it more easily. Castor oil is similarly double the dose for an average size dog: give two dessertspoons with some honey to make it palatable.

Following the strong purge, now employ the well-proved virus killing herbs which were formerly used to combat 'plagues'. These are garlic, wormwood, southernwood, sage, rue, rosemary. Give either finely minced and mixed into pills by blending with flour and honey, or in a prepared tablet form of reliable make. An average dose would be two tea-spoons of the hand-mixed pills or two or three tablets of the herbal formula, given morning and night throughout the illness.

Another typical and dangerous symptom of CPV is the rapid dehydration which in itself can prove a quick killer. Dehydration can be treated orally, the more stressful vascular treatment is not essential. In fact the BBC, in their World Service 'Science in Action' programmes, have often talked about a 'saviour' tea which is used to help save the lives of infants in Third World lands where dysentery is a typical and widespread killer. The 'tea' is merely fresh water, fortified with a pinch of salt and a larger amount of glucose, fed to the infants at frequent intervals while the diarrhoea runs itself clean. The same treatment for puppies: frequent dosing, at three-hourly intervals, with saviour tea but with improvements to that advised for human infants. Use barley water instead of plain water and make the barley water with a strong solution of sage tea. An extra benefit is then added by the use of honey instead of just glucose and salt. Honey itself is a life-giver and heart strengthener and it can be digested easily by the bloodstream. The exact formula to every table-spoon measure is: into the barley and sage water add one level teaspoon of pure honey, one of glucose, and half, or less, of a small teaspoon of sea salt. If the salt is ejected, then use less. The tea should be an internal soother and fortifier; an emetic is not required.

To prevent the painful vomiting which is a distressing symptom of CPV, make pills of grated gentian root. About a teaspoonful should be sufficient to ease the vomiting. Make gentian pills with flour and honey or give the gentian in a spoonful of milk.

Dr Richard Pitcairn gives the original advice, of which I thoroughly approve, that severe dehydration can also be given immediate help by feeding liquids through the other end of the animal, the anus. The same mineral-rich, anti-dehydration mixture as I have suggested for oral use can also be given by enema into the lower bowel from where it is quickly absorbed by the body. Do not use a complicated tubing enema; the simple bulb type is best here. Merely raise the hindquarters of the dog or cat, insert the end of the enema tube, then slowly press on the bulb to inject the contents into the bowel. Keep the hindquarters raised for several minutes to prevent the fluid from running back and out through the anus.

After several days of anti-dehydration treatment, when the bad odour has left the diarrhoea, soothe the stomach and intestinal tract by giving drinks of such long-proved beneficial and strengthening natural substances as slippery- (red) elm bark, arrowroot, marshmallow root, crushed dill seed and barley flour made into a gruel by adding milk and honey. NR formula gruel has all these ingredients and it is advisable to keep some always on hand in case of dysentery emergencies. It is also a great and very strengthening weaning formula and is excellent for the in-whelp and nursing bitch.

Further to save life, do remember the general, sensible, 'old-fashioned' care of all sick creatures, be they human or animal: a well-shaded, airy and totally quiet sickroom; isolation from fellow creatures which may disturb sleep (vitally needed for recovery); fresh drinking water at all times with a little wine vinegar or cider vinegar added, a teaspoon to a pint of water.

For my writings on the clinical experiences of my own Turkuman Afghans and the experience of others, plus homeopathic advice for CPV, there are details in my recently published book, *Three Virus Ailments of the Modern Dog* (obtainable from NR Products suppliers).

PIGMENTATION, FAULTY   Many dogs suffer from faulty pigmentation; this is especially true of specific breeds, and notably the imported ones.

The most usual body parts for faulty pigmentation are nose, eye rims, toenails. Light noses, however, should not be penalized in the imported breeds during the winter months, for very often such is but the protective snow-blending colour of Nature, e.g. Samoyeds (Arctic); Afghans, light-coated (Afghanistan); Finnish spitz (Finland); golden retrievers and borzois (Russia), may all quite correctly develop light noses during those months when their native countries would be expecting snow.

Treatment   Where pigmentation is truly faulty, the quickest and well-proved remedy is seaweed, given in powder form, increasing by twice the normal daily tonic dose of seaweed. It is outstanding for the dark pigment that it produces. Also helpful are: finely chopped watercress and mustard and cress, molasses, grape juice, raisins.

PNEUMONIA, PLEURISY, BRONCHITIS   These lung ailments are often a complication of distemper. A typical pneumonia case will be seen breathing rapidly, with mouth kept closed; eyes will be bloodshot, fever high.

These ailments properly treated can be cured as surely as canine distemper, and likewise usually run a course of three weeks.

Treatment   A first need is strict fasting in order to cleanse the body of accumulated toxins. It is the strenous cleansing efforts of the body which are the main cause of the very high fever found in canine lung disorders and which are not an unfavourable condition. Commenting on fever, the great Greek doctor, Hippocrates, said: 'Give me a high fever and I can cure the ailment', meaning that the heat of fever burns up harmful bacteria.

Second need is the use of antiseptic herbs, especially garlic and eucalyptus. The action of garlic on the lungs is a remarkable one: it has been praised throughout the ages as a tuberculosis cure, and even in this modern time of artificial chemical medicine it is given credit as such. Recently the daily papers have published reports of work done by the Russian, Professor Thokin, of Toms University, in regard to tuberculosis, he having prepared a serum from onions and garlic which will kill tuberculosis bacilli after only five minutes' treatment. (At last the production of a harmless serum! And one not derived from the body fluids of artificially diseased and tortured animals.)

Third, there comes the strengthening and soothing of the body, especially the nerves, through the feeding of that miraculous product of Nature – honey – which substance, in pneumonia treatment, even at a time of high fever, can be made into honey balls and fed to the dog or pushed down the throat; the honey will give great relief to the inflamed throat. Three drops of oil of eucalyptus can be added twice daily to the honey balls. Finally, the provision of abundant fresh air, which is as essential to a pneumonia case as is water to a gastritis case, although orthodox medicine usually places more importance on much stuffy warmth than on fresh air. And the orthodox, in order to keep the sick dog 'warm and free from draughts' – being the way in which that common ruling is usually expressed – keep windows closed, and the dog is thereby ignorantly, and cruelly, deprived of the air which its panting lungs crave. The nasal passages can be kept open by the use of inhalants such as eucalyptus, camphor, thyme, in form of essential oils. All are rather strong for the dog, therefore use only one or two drops mixed well into lanoline and then pressed up the nostrils. These oils are very effective in cases of congested lungs. The throat and chest should then be frictioned with a lotion of one teaspoon eucalyptus to two tablespoons water. A few drops of eucalyptus can also be given twice daily on a small piece of cube sugar or on honey, pushed down the throat. The throat and chest area will also benefit from massage with Vicks Vapo-rub or Tiger Balm.

Having given an outline of things to do in pneumonia treatment, I must mention a few of the things *not* to do. First, the rigid avoidance of all chemical drugs, especially those of the sulphonamide group. The rapid 'cure' that such drugs often produce is no real cure, it is merely suppression of the symptoms of pneumonia through violent interference of the drug in the body's cleansing efforts; such false healing provides ideal soil for the breeding, later, of tubercular bacteria. (Note present-day tuberculosis increase.) Second, the refraining from giving all the usual stimulants so commonly prescribed in the treatment of pneumonia.

An excellent medicine is made from the skins of washed lemons, three lemons to one and a half pints cold water. Bring to boil for three minutes. Some needles of the common pine-tree, the buds, are also very helpful, one teaspoonful added to the lemon brew. When cooled to tepid, restore the juice of the lemons. Sweeten with one tablespoon honey. Add two inches solid stick Spanish liquorice; dissolve well. The liquorice dissolved in this brew will then have its medicinal properties further enhanced. Also thick, pure honey rolled into balls and placed in the mouth or pressed down the throat gives nourishment, removes throat soreness and, like the liquorice, produces expectoration.

In the treatment kennel the air can be kept sweet and moist by using a steam kettle, a few drops of such a substance as eucalyptus oil, or Vapex, being added to each pint of water poured into the kettle. The freshening effect this has on the atmosphere is remarkable, and is highly appreciated by the dog. Elecampane herb and pine needles can also be used for inhalation by steam vapour.

The mouth and throat should be cleansed three times daily

with lemon water, also the nose thoroughly washed or syringed out with the lemon water, while the body must be internally disinfected with garlic, which exerts a remarkable healing effect on the mucous membranes. Alternatively use Herbal Compound tablets.

If this treatment is carried out faithfully, the dog will remain strong and will be found to be easily cured of this complication. But if the treatment is not fully and sufficiently followed, then there is a danger of the dread oedema of the lungs, brought about by the weakening of the heart on its left side and its subsequent failure to drive the venous blood through the lungs. Blood-filled fluid begins to pass through the nostrils, 'squelching' sounds can be heard in the lungs, and death takes place, the blood then flowing out through the mouth.

Let me repeat, such a happening is unusual, and is very rare if the case has been correctly treated.

Note: A dog with complications of the lungs *craves* fresh air. Fresh air at such a time is of far greater importance than food.

POISONING The commonest poisons with which a dog is likely to come into contact are as follows (their neutralizing agents – antidotes – are bracketed with them): strychnine – in vermin exterminators – (permanganate of potash in solution, about a saltspoon to half a pint of tepid water); phosphorus – in rat poison, matchheads – (soda water and milk of magnesia); crude stove paraffin (stiff dose of salad oil to mix with the paraffin and cause its removal through the bowels); white lead – from paint, etc – (Epsom salts in solution, about one teaspoon to one cupful tepid water).

Treatment The general treatment is the same for all poisons, with the exception of strychnine, only differing in the antidotes to be used. First there must be rapid removal of all possible poison by the aid of an emetic, the best of which is a piece of washing soda, the size of a penny for an average size dog, pushed well down the throat; this will induce almost immediate vomiting. Failing soda, common salt should be used, a stiff dose of two teaspoons in a small cupful of water being the general dose. A strong infusion of radish is also an emetic. Another useful treatment to induce rapid vomiting is a strong solution of mustard powder in warm water: a heaped dessertspoon of table mustard powder mixed into liquid form with warm water. After the emetic has been given, the next principle is laxative treatment to clear the bowels of the poison.

The best treatment is drenching with one of the natural aperient waters; failing this, then *senna* must be made quickly (there being no time for making by the better, cold-water-soaking method) by scalding about seven pods with boiling water, allowing to stand for a few minutes, then crushing the pods to extract all moisture and reducing to blood heat by the addition of a little cold water. The dog must then be fasted for at least two to three days to allow the body, freed from the task of food digestion, to exert all of its energies on the removal of the irritant poisons, and also in the mere main-tenance of life. Laxatives should be given night and morning, and the antidotes should be discontinued after the first day. The fast should be one of water only. If the dog has retained life up to the third day, then healing treatment can be com-menced.

Whether a dog is to live or to die, following intake of poison, largely depends on the dog's previous health record. A well-reared healthy animal will have great natural reserves of body energy with which to expel the poison from the body; there will also be no danger of heart failure, which is the commonest cause of death in poisoning cases. Honey should be given from the very first hour of poisoning, for its heart and nerve restorative properties, also laxative and alkaline properties, internal healing powers, are all of the greatest value. Lumps of thick honey, about the size of a hazel-nut – average dose – should be pushed down the throat many times a day during the first stages of treatment. Give fresh milk (not Long-life) to neutralize poison.

Following the fast, a recuperative diet should consist of three meals per day of one cupful of slippery elm food (tree-barks' gruel) mixed with honey and milk. More can be given if the dog appears hungry: three to four cupfuls of the mixture for a large size dog, as required. The slippery elm acts as an internal poultice, soothing and healing the inflamed lining of stomach and intestines. After an average of three days on such a fluid diet, the fluid can be thickened with flaked barley for the midday and evening meals, but no other food should be given for at least seven days, as the body will be in no fit state to deal with other foods. I should mention the use, also, of my own formula medicine, the leaf-plasma tablets, which are highly alkaline in their action, and are so wonderfully nerve restorative.

There is one thing of special importance in phosphorus poisoning (which poisoning may well be caused through the eating of matchheads – a common habit in young puppies – or from rat and mice exterminators): all fats must be withheld during treatment, in order to keep extra work from the liver which is the organ most usually affected in this type of poisoning, and fats are also an extra-harmful mixture with phosphorus. All milk given must be skimmed. In phosphorus poisoning the dog develops an ungovernable thirst, the intake of water each time being followed by severe vomiting which is very exhausting. However, I am of the opinion that it is wrong to withhold water, and at the usual meal hours, three times daily, the dog should be allowed to drink its fill of water. Rue is an ancient and famed poison antidote.

The plant is crushed and rolled into pills.

An infusion of hyssop plant given morning and evening is highly effective as a remedial agent in all forms of poisoning. Foxes are said to seek out this plant when poisoned. Neat witch hazel, a tablespoon three times daily, given with the hyssop, and given alone at midday, is invaluable on account of its healing powers.

I have had two experiences of severe poisoning among my own Afghan hounds; in both cases very large amounts of poison were taken. The first case was an Afghan bitch, given a half-pint drench of stove paraffin in error, from a bottle which should by rights have held aperient water. Treated as instructed above, she fully recovered in ten days and has had perfect health ever since (this was the Best-in-Show winning bitch, Turkuman Wild Kashmiri Iris). The second case was of phosphorus rat-poisoning in an Afghan dog. Many pieces of bread spread thickly with rat poison had been eaten. The dog was the equally well-known Turkuman Mogul Rose-tree; no one thought he could recover.

I feel strongly that the making of phosphorus vermin poisons should be prohibited, that terrible internal burning is too cruel even for the vermin for which they are intended. Vermin-poisons manufacturers should be made to witness animals in the terrible death throes from their products.

Strychnine is a peril to dogs, cats and wild birds, not only because it lies around in meat baited for vermin extermination and is used for foxes in poisoned poultry, but also because it is the poison chosen for feeding to off-leash dogs by members of sanitary departments, who will feed poisoned meat to any dog which they select, even if that dog carries a number disc showing that it has been vaccinated according to their petty and unhealthy laws. As with the other poisons, give an immediate emetic then, if the poison has already circulated in the system of the dog, an artificially imposed stupor is the only hope of saving the case, because the nervous spasms brought on by strychnine will cause death through heart failure, Get veterinary surgery help immediately for the sleep. An injection of a quarter grain of morphia for an average size dog should be given hypodermically at intervals, to maintain the stupor until the spasms and the rigidity caused have decreased. The animal must be kept in complete seclusion and quiet, and in a darkened room, for the narcotics to be effective. Noise and the alarm and grief of the owners of the poisoned dog are greatly magnified to the animal under narcotic treatment who is under such tension, distress and suffering pain, and the disturbance will increase the severity of these spasms. Put cold vinegar-soaked cloths on the head, and hot bottles at the feet (and also pray to Saint Francis, patron saint of all animals, and to God for the dog's recovery). Give also charcoal tablets, famed for absorbing poisons, two tablets nightly for average size dog. Make sure tablets are true vegetable charcoal and not made from bone charcoal.

An old, but excellent, remedy is egg whites, which take the burn out of scalds and burns and cool the chemical fire of poison. For dog or cat, whites of three eggs, well whipped, then poured into the mouth.

Always seek veterinary aid speedily. Tranquillizers and anaesthetics are valuable help.

RABIES Fortunately rabies is not very widespread: it can and has been cured frequently, as can well be proved by reading old documents concerning this disease. It has always been an uncommon ailment and remains so to this day. I must stress that the fear of rabies is much fostered by the makers of rabies vaccines, used in so-called prevention and in treatment of human cases who have had contact with rabies but have not actually been bitten by a rabid animal. There are

lurid posters around to spread rabies fear and rabies vaccination is imposed by law on millions of dogs worldwide who
are *never* likely to have any contact whatsoever with rabies
and whose health is greatly undermined by this annual dose
of real poison. I have avoided such vaccination absolutely for
my own dogs and I hope that one day such a commercialized
infringement of personal liberties will be banned by the
power of public opinion.

Symptoms Strangely, they are very similar to canine parvovirus in their first stages: the symptoms are related to water.
The alternative name for rabies is hydrophobia, which
means water phobia, fixation or fear. First there is a mad
desire to drink and then comes a sustained longing to drink
but a terror of the very sight of water. A rabid creature will
stand by water, foaming at the mouth and uttering terrible-
to-hear screams or growls, and prevented by the final water
phobia from satisfying its, by then, raging thirst. Brain control finally snaps and the rabies case loses all self-control and
rushes round biting at everything in a sort of mad self-
protection bid, until finally the heart collapses from the
extreme exhaustion of the biting fury and merciful death
comes, unless the rabid creature can be stopped earlier by
shooting.

The development of the water fear (the final stage of the
rabies illness) may take many weeks if the victim is of fairly
strong constitution. Throughout those weeks there is great
thirst, but the water is not retained. Rarely it is vomited up,
but more typically it pours from the bowels, foamy and putrid, similar to that which occurs in CPV. There is the same
CPV abnormal look in the eyes and the same rapid and
intense dehydration.

Treatment Unfortunately, in most countries of the world
where rabies is known to exist, dog and cat owners are not

allowed to treat rabies if it should develop. No matter how beloved is the dog or cat concerned, immediate death by injection or shooting is enforced. Fortunately, when I treated three cases of rabies I did not know what illness I was treating; I considered the symptoms to indicate a form of poisoning. Not until the last case manifested all the rage symptoms of the disease did I know that I had true rabies on my premises and had been luckily saved by herbal treatment of two of my cases (both Afghan hounds) from the development of the disease into its final stage. That could have meant that my two big and very powerful male Afghans would have been running amok in the madness of hydrophobia and could have killed me and others. The dogs had been infected by contact only, not by bite, from a wolfdog brought back from Syria by an Israeli soldier, and I was able to treat them successfully. One, in fact, was back to normal health in a week and suffered no dehydration. The third case, a Pekinese and not NR at all, developed total dehydration and had to be destroyed.

Further information about rabies, including more clinical experience, can be found in my book, *Three Virus Ailments of the Modern Dog*.

RHEUMATISM In damp climates rheumatism is a quite frequent ailment of dogs, especially aged ones. Only the dampness is not wholly responsible: the body first has to be in an unhealthy state to produce this condition of rheumatism or arthritis. A tendency to joint ailments also can be inherited but, as with most hereditary ailments, can be bred out by Natural Rearing. Canine rheumatism is found most frequently in shoulders and chest, or back and loins – where it is called lumbago. The feet are sometimes affected. In the limbs lameness often develops. The only certain preventive of rheumatism is: correct rearing on a raw foods diet, with provision of good, dry housekeeping, and especially the avoidance of sour, urine-saturated kennel runs, also providing all the sunlight that the dogs themselves desire.

Internal Treatment Internal cleansing with antiseptic herbs, especially garlic; honey is also an important remedy, its alkaline properties reducing the acid deposits of rheumatism. An infusion of parsley leaves, or fed raw, finely minced, is excellent, especially when the ailment is chronic. Parsley alone has cured even severe cases of rheumatism and arthritis. Also give as much nettle as possible, for above all other plants it has the power to dissolve uric acid crystals and therefore gives much relief in rheumatic ailments. Nettles should be gathered with scissors, as the leafage stings the hands, then plunged into boiling water for a few minutes, using very little water; they are then ready for use, mixed into the cereal feed. I have prepared tablets of nettle with seaweed and comfrey. Comfrey is a proved remedy for rheumatism and arthritis. Also feed minced watercress and other cresses, and minced onion and garlic greens.

External Treatment Massage with lotion made from an infusion of seaweed and thyme, equal parts, standard infusion. Apply warm. Give also, on the meat, finely chopped green leaves of celery, also a dessertspoon of celery seed. Miss D. Mills, The Kennels, Dawlish, Devon, reported: 'I have cured an Irish Setter – after only three weeks' treatment – of prolonged and acute rheumatism, by your herbal treatment. The dog was so ill he could not stand and the orthodox treatment could do nothing more for him.'

RINGWORM This fungus disease is distinguished by circular patches on any part of the body, often on the face. The hair falls. It is contagious.

Treatment Treat as for mange if widespread. If merely in several patches a speedy cure can be obtained by dressing with pure, fresh-squeezed lemon juice. This forms a glaze over the skin surface and ringworm, being a fungus type of parasite, is suffocated and withers. The glaze given by fingernail varnish can also be used. This likewise prevents the fungus from breathing.

RUBARTH DISEASE (This is contagious hepatitis; see Hepatitis.)

SCALDS Many small dogs, especially toys and terrier breeds, get under the feet of their owners when they are carrying boiling water, and get badly scalded. I learnt a burns-scalds treatment from peasants of the Sierra Nevada mountains, Spain, which gives remarkable results. Bathe the injured area first with pure vinegar, then spread honey thickly over the area, ten minutes later. Keep applying dressings of honey until all burning pain ceases, then bandage lightly with cotton cloths over a dressing of honey to exclude air. Long-haired dogs must be clipped before applying the honey: they would lose their burnt or scalded hair anyway. If the dog tries to tear off the bandaging, he must wear a broad collar of cardboard to restrict movement of his head. Another excellent and proved burns-scalds remedy is raw potato. Wash and crush raw potato and apply the juicy pulp to the area, or the potato can be finely grated on a metal grater and the juice expressed by pressing through cheesecloth. Then if none of these remedies is available, there is a cure learnt from the natives of Hawaii. Place the injured area under tepid water, and keep under water, excluding all air, for at least one hour, until the burning pain ceases. Application of egg whites is also curative.

SCURF   Presence of much scurf indicates excess mucus in the system. Also lack of exercise in fresh air will create greasy skin and thus scurf, and lack of sufficient oil in the diet.

Treatment   This is both internal and external. Internal is dependent on diet. Cut down on milk and starches. Give daily a small teaspoon of oil of sesame, sunflower or corn. Feed cooked, minced carrot, minced watercress. Externally friction with a brew of meadowsweet or rosemary. Also the hair treatment for Baldness (see this chapter) can be used with advantage.

SEASON, DELAYED OR FAULTY   (See Streptococcal Infection) The simple cleansing treatment for 'strep' will restore normality to the reproductive organs. But it is necessary to advise that bitches of some breeds, especially the Oriental ones such as Afghans, salukis, and chows, are often only once yearly in season when in normal health. Give raspberry leaves, raw and minced, mixed with food, as an infusion or in tablet form; natural vitamins C and E; minced raw pumpkin seeds.

SENILITY   Senility in the dog and cat (also in humans) is caused largely by the daily feeding of cooked foods in place of the natural raw, and by lack of sufficient running exercise, causing the blood to lack oxygen and also the lungs and heart to degenerate. Today many dogs are declining in health from the age of seven years, and most of them have disordered kidneys from that age onward. In the old days when dog rearing was more natural, dogs remained in good health up to twenty years of age. I have met a number of dogs of such age owned by desert-roaming Bedouin Arabs and by Spanish peasants. In Granada, Spain, a market-stall holder had a spaniel aged twenty-four years, and Sunny Shay, Grandeur

Afghans, New York, kept her Afghan, Champion Taj Akbaruu of Grandeur, to the age of twenty-two.

After fifteen years of NR in Switzerland, Miss Marjorie Pickance, La Tour de Peilz, Ct Vaud, owner of the Kentony Pekinese, known throughout Switzerland for their great health (now retired from showing and breeding), writes to me:

I have two stud dogs who are thirteen and look and behave as if they were about six, and a bitch of nearly fifteen. All are a tremendous credit to NR. Most of the others are over ten. All these dogs are in wonderful condition and coat and seem to enjoy every minute of the day and every meal. No need to coax any of them to eat, we have always kept strictly to NR diet.

Saluki champion Knightellington Vandal won Best-in-Show at the Saluki Club Show of England, when aged nearly ten years. Saved by herbal medicine when his life was despaired of, he was reared and is owned by the Misses Kean and Mackenzie, at their Ajman Kennels, Oxford. Country dogs, living free, unchained, hunting around, are notable for long life, as likewise are the dogs of gypsies and wandering Bedouins of the Arab lands. Such people commonly own two dogs who live into their twentieth year and over, horses (and camels) of these natural people likewise are exceptionally long lived. The United States Ch. Turkuman Nissim's Laurel, exported from my Turkuman Afghan kennel to Sol. M. Malkin and Sunny Shay, Grandeur Afghans, lived to the age of sixteen years, siring champions when aged fourteen, and winning Hound Groups when turned twelve years.

For longevity for *all* dogs, feed a raw foods diet, as Nature intended for the dog, fox, wolf, etc. (Some wolves in the wild, recognizable by their battle scars by those who have seen them on the Turkish hills, attain thirty years of age.)

248

Provide also sunlight and free-running exercise and access to wild medicinal herbs, then long life will be your dog's heritage.

SHOCK   When a dog or cat is suffering from shock, resulting from severe wounds in a fight or from car or other accidents, do not give solid food for twenty-four hours at least; give instead a teaspoon of pure honey, liquefied by stirring in a half teaspoon of brandy or sweet red wine, and give three times daily. Then restore to normal food, beginning with one day on fluid milk-honey only. Give also rock-rose as a strong brew, or bee-balm (*Melissa*). Dr Bach's Floral Remedies supply a preparation of rock-rose (from herbal shops). Elder-blossom tea or elderberry wine are of long-proved help.

SICKNESS, AND PROLONGED VOMITING   As with diarrhoea, sickness in the dog is usually either a rapid, natural cleansing of the body or a mere symptom of some other ailment: distemper, leptospirosis, hepatitis, parvovirus (see treatments, this chapter). Deliberate sickness is produced in the dog by the eating of couch grass, which acts as an internal rake, scraping out mucus-embedded impurities. Prolonged frothy, yellow sickness needs treatment to sweeten the digestive system, and vomiting of food needs immediate fasting.

Treatment   Herbs to sweeten a sour digestive tract, cause of prolonged sickness, are peppermint, rosemary, thyme, plus tablets of vegetable charcoal. Make infusion of one or another of these herbs, and give to the fasting dog – dose, two tablespoons three times daily. In the dangerous vomiting of Stuttgart disease, parvovirus and some other ailments, grate raw gentian root preferably, or buy the powdered root. Roll the grated gentian into pills the size of a garden pea, using a mass of thick honey and flour to bind it. An average dog

249

would require approximately twelve pills for a day's treatment. Fast the dog on lemon barley water during the gentian treatment. If gentian is not available then try and get the more common St John's wort as a tea, fortified with peppermint.

Bitches in sound health often suffer from a slight nervous sickness during the first few weeks of the in-whelp period. This does not indicate ill health; merely give infusion of raspberry leaves and two or three charcoal tablets morning and night.

There is also sickness caused by nervous excitability, travel by car, ship, or plane. The greyhound breeds seem to be the most frequent sufferers from travel sickness. Animals prone to such sickness should be fasted for at least twelve hours before long journeys. At the time of travel they should be given balls of thick honey, into which a little powdered ginger has been mixed, pressed down their throats; honey will settle the stomach nerves; or yet a better remedy is to mix tree-barks' flour and powdered ginger into the honey, one small teaspoon of flour and a pinch of ginger to one heaped tablespoon thick honey. Dogs travel best on car floors rather than seats if they are bad travellers; however, car floors cannot be used during hot weather as they heat up and are harmful then to health.

SORE PADS, SPLIT PADS, ETC Concrete roads, gravel paths, and flinty hillsides often injure the foot pads of dogs when they take much exercise over such surfaces. The normal surface for the dog is earth – grasslands, sands, or rocks. The dogs of heavy build, such as Great Danes, Irish wolfhounds, Newfoundlands, etc, are the most prone to this trouble. Generally bad feet are also a sign of health decline; and attention, therefore, should be given to the diet, especially if the dog is overweight.

Treatment   Rest the dog from all exercise or work for several days, at least until the splits in the pads close up. Bathe the pads three times daily with a lotion made from boiled potato peelings, a very large handful of peelings to one quart cold water, brought to a boil and simmered for ten minutes. Do not strain. Deep fissures should be treated with swabs of cotton soaked in a lotion made from ivy leaves. To every cupful of the ivy, add one dessertspoon of witch hazel. A dusting with fine oatmeal completes the treatment. At night soak the feet in castor oil and tie on cloths.

SPRAINS   These are usually caused by running over hard land, especially land rutted by ploughing, or landing badly from a high jump. With a sprain the dog limps badly and swelling often occurs.

Treatment   Resting and application of cold-water and vinegar cloths around the limb. An old and effective horse remedy is to apply a paste made from whitening (whitewash) and cow dung. Spread thickly around the affected area and bandage lightly. The herbal remedies are comfrey or mallow. Make a standard infusion of either herb and bathe the injured area before applying bandages. Dog owners who live by the sea can stand the injured dog in the sea, or put the limb in a bucket of sea water for ten minutes or so. This is a very simple and effective cure, much used for valuable race-horses.

STERILITY   Animals which are habitually sterile may well be carriers of streptococcal bacteria or of leptospirosis or hepatitis. But mention should be made of the effect of diet on fertility. Modern diet greatly lacks the fertility vitamins, which are removed in modern milling, especially vitamins B and E. Sterility may also be caused by obesity (which see).

Also the unnatural isolation of the sexes – no access to communal mixing will cause frigidity.

Treatment Place all sterile animals on a natural raw foods diet (see NR diet, Chapter 1). Give leaf-extract tablets containing seaweed, nettle, etc, also wheat-germ flakes and raw eggs. Some natural, herbal aphrodisiacs are bee-balm, mint (especially wild water mint), and the aromatics, thyme, marjoram, sage, and fennel. All should be given very finely chopped on the raw meat. Honey also aids fertility, and young maize (corn) cobs, given raw, grated on a vegetable grater. Grated raw almonds are a splendid fertility aid, especially for male animals; mix the almonds with the cereal; also, raw eggs. Feed liquorice to females.

STINGS Dogs are apt to snap at bees, wasps and hornets, or they tread on such insects, and in consequence get stung. Stings on the limbs are treated by application of a layer of whitewash, after removing the sting if it can be found. The whitewash should be removed after half an hour. Or put on lemon juice, or vinegar, garlic or onion juice, or a thick paste of either mud and water or common salt and water, bound into place. For stings in the mouth five drinks of milk with a little wine added; without food for one day or more, until swelling subsides.

STREPTOCOCCAL INFECTION The one and only cause of streptococcal infections and losses, as with distemper, is faulty rearing and over-commercialism. I have often given the opinion that a large percentage of present-day dog breeders would happily feed their dogs on a diet of sawdust if they could get away with it!

The wish for cheap, quickly prepared foods and medicines, and utter neglect of kennel hygiene, with horrible overcrowding, sour earth and urine-soaked wooden buildings typify dog rearing today in most countries, and dogs will continue to suffer from 'plague' diseases until the simple laws of natural, clean, and kindly dog rearing become common to the majority of kennels. Nature Rearing has already been put into worldwide practice, and in kennels where once not a single litter had been reared in years, now litters are being reared easily, the stock showing a high standard of health. I have also met with many modern dog keepers who allege that they are rearing on natural, healthful lines, but who are continuing to keep their stock overcrowded and under-exercised: not all the medicines – herbal or otherwise – or the most perfect of diets will be able to maintain normal health in such cases. I am not at all impressed with kennels keeping anything over twenty dogs. I cannot understand the mentality of such kennel owners. Is it that they think that in having large numbers the law of averages makes the breeding of a champion the more certain? But how different are the true facts as to the breeding of champions: again and again it will be found that it is the 'little' kennel owner who breeds the champions, and the other 'big' kennels which buy up their winning stock – and often lose through disease, latent in their kennels, the new-purchased stock.

It will be appropriate here to quote from a remarkable agricultural booklet, sent to me by one of my veterinary clients, Miss C.D. Wilson, of Ludlow, and which upholds in every instance all that I have been stating and writing for so many years on the subject of canine rearing and medicine. It is *Re-Fertilization of a Large Wiltshire Farm by Compost*, by F. Sykes, also author of *Modern Humus Farming* and *Food, Farming and the Future* (Faber and Faber). He stresses that healthy soil is the root of all health and of disease prevention and cure, that all chemicals both in soil treatment and food materials should be strictly avoided, and likewise use of all vaccine and similar remedies. A case is quoted of a thorough-bred mare which developed contagious abortion, and whose destruction was advised by an 'eminent veterinarian'; the mare was subjected to natural medicine methods and made a perfect recovery (typical of numerous cases of streptococcal infection in bitches, which cases, removed to clean kennel runs [grass sown], correctly dieted, sufficiently exercised, have made perfect recoveries and have whelped and nursed perfectly normal litters, the puppies of which have grown up into disease-free adults – this, from bitches tested for presence of b.h.s., and found to be 'infected'). He writes:

> . . . our most valuable thoroughbred mare contracted the dangerous disease – contagious abortion. An eminent veterinarian advised her destruction. I declined the advice and determined a treatment of my own, which was to turn the mare out into a large paddock where no horse stock had been grazed, where artificial manures had never been used, and where she was condemned to live for two years eating practically nothing but grass. At the end of this period she was examined by a competent vet and declared clean. She was mated and artificially inseminated; she later proved in foal, and subsequently bred over the next seven years four valuable foals, she herself living to the ripe old age of 21 years. Here was my first attempt to cure an allegedly incurable disease by giving the creature nothing but grass-grown land where artificial manures had never been applied, in other words Nature's food from humus-filled land.

The writer then goes on to describe how large-scale disease came to the farm (through the usual causes which are the same source of disease in dog kennels). Again I quote from this booklet:

We bought valuable cattle and put them on land which was couch-ridden and very infertile, and the ability of which to sustain life was so low that food of every kind had to be brought from elsewhere to augment the supply of the poor herbage. The heavy stocking and treading began to develop other troubles and, as always on dirty, foul, neglected land, disease of every kind began to show itself in the cattle to the pre-war value of over £2,000. The veterinary service could help us but little. As is usual, the course followed had to be devised by the farmer. We decided to plough up the whole 750 acres. We determined to try now home-grown food, especially avoiding all factory compound foods and concentrates. Above all to apply artificials nowhere. And after seven years of heart-breaking toil, with the added difficulties of war-time (1) completely rid the farm of disease; (2) built up a large herd of home-bred, attested dairy cattle, tubercle-free for over three years now, and of a soundness of constitution to all critical appearances such that no expert would believe that any scourge had ever visited the farm, and (3) as each succeeding generation of young stock is born we have unmistakable evidence of still greater stamina and endurance.

The (3) result is of special importance to dog breeders, for likewise in dog breeding, with each generation of Natural Reared stock improved health is a natural and positive result – greater size, bone, hair growth, and general disease resistance.

Concerning all this, Mrs Doxford, the cocker spaniel judge and breeder, Broomleaf Cockers, Ewshot, Surrey, has reported:

I am rearing my fifth generation of NR – Natural Reared – stock now; and their disease resistance is amazing, as is their growth and condition. What I think is even more satisfactory (to both you and me) is that young stock sold from these kennels have come through epidemics in their new owners' kennels, *unscathed*; whereas the other stock has succumbed; the other stock of course not having been reared by natural methods.

In the summing-up of his leaflet, Mr Sykes, concerning disease prevention and the appalling record of disease rife in the world today, writes:

Then is there no hope for mankind? Yes, there is one hope – disease. It may teach us the mistakes we should avoid. The continued use of artificials is the first mistake, for it produces food of diminishingly efficient feeding value for both man and beast, and is reducing vitality so low that resistance to the malign bacteria of disease is becoming less. Notwithstanding, the Ministry of Health can be liquidated in a very short time. The second mistake is the feeding of concentrated cakes and meals, the by-products of the soap and oil industries – yet more of the powerful vested interests. They are unnatural foods and are fed to cattle and poultry to stimulate the production of unnatural quantities of meat, milk, eggs, and poultry meat. I have cured disease in animals by cutting-out the feeding of factory-made concentrates and substituting such foods as oats, peas, beans, and grass, grown on the farm on humus-sufficient fertile land.

Here should be mentioned that the by-products of soap and other industries are in use also in the canine world. The dried meat in use in popular dog foods is often the residue from soap factories, animal material from which all fat has been extracted by means of caustics, in soap manufacture – the harmfulness of such 'food' to the canine stomach and intestines can well be imagined. To continue from the agricultural treatise:

Two difficulties presented themselves. (1) Farmers will not

cease to use artificial fertilizers for their land, because they have been taught by clever propaganda over a long period of time, that it is more profitable to use them for crop production than keeping and relying upon livestock . . . (2) Farmers will continue the use of factory concentrates for their cattle feeding, because again skilled propaganda has driven into their heads that they can produce neither milk nor meat without them. It does not begin to occur to one farmer in a thousand that the prevalence of contagious abortion, turbercular and other ills of their livestock may be brought about by the use of artificials on the land, or the use of the concentrated cakes fed to cows . . . And so disease will come. Come? It is already here, everywhere in abundance. There are few disease-free herds in this country. Foot-and-mouth is periodically rampant; tuberculosis is as common as the dawn of day; Johne's disease and barrenness are rife everywhere. It is estimated on reliable data that eighty per cent of dairy cattle passing through the market are diseased in one way or another. The milking life of the average cow is now reduced to two and a half years. Is the Ministry of Agriculture worried? Yes, indeed they are. Remedies? Oh, yes, vaccines and veterinary panels. But why not start at the bottom, in the soil itself? Hush! No one has ever thought of that. *In officialdom you must never go to the root cause of disease. That is a most unprofessional approach'* [the italics are mine].

As in agriculture, the canine world is faced with misleading propaganda largely sponsored by vaccine and chemical manufacturers, and the equally mischievous advertising of the Department of Health, with its stress on the importance of diphtheria inoculation and the 'fine' results obtained (such propaganda is becoming increasingly necessary because members of the armed forces in World War II, having witnessed the deleterious effect of army vaccinations on their own health, are insisting that their children be kept free of such unhygienic and unnatural practices).

Then, as with the farmers, there is the laziness of dog breeders. Correct rearing takes much time. In natural diet alone it requires far more care and thought than the general orthodox feeding method – a method which is fit only for the raising of those fat semi-diseased beasts, swine – of over-boiling supplies of meat, pouring the resultant liquid over white hound meal and its percentage of soap-factory by-product meat fibre, and feeding both meat and greasy white-cereal biscuit together at one meal, and expecting good health to result! (Little wonder that tapeworm remedies are in great demand, and eczema and hysteria cures!)

Proper feeding takes much care and time and planning; the preparation of the daily ration for each dog, of raw finely chopped green food – a health essential – takes time; the herbs have to be gathered, let alone prepared for use. Raw meat takes longer to cut up than cooked – for the latter is partly disintegrated flesh; the whole-grain cereal dishes need careful preparation; and ample supply of fresh unpasteurized milk is required – dried milk, in place of fresh, is one of the most deadly foods offered to dogs, and especially to young puppies. That is why I state emphatically that it is not pos-sible for good health to be maintained in any kennel where the number of inmates is overlarge. Cattle can be kept in herds of fair size: they get most of their own foods through grazing – it is merely necessary to ensure that their pasture is healthy. But the dogs must have all of their food fed to them by man – except for the occasional rabbit which they may take themselves. Furthermore, dogs quickly foul and sour the premises where they are kept and the ground on which they take exercise – cattle are mainly beneficial to the land. *Over-crowding, wrong feeding, neglectful rearing – especially where suf-ficient exercise is concerned – use of chemicals and vaccines in canine medicine, with subsequent health degenerations, are the root causes of present-day prevalence of canine b.h.s. disease.* The remedy for its prevention and cure lies in the hands of the breeders.

And now to go on to streptococcal disease itself. It is absurd to take the mere presence of streptococcal bacteria as being proof of the presence of the disease, especially when it should be remembered that streptococcal bacteria are among the most widely distributed and the most common of all bacteria of the body, and are to be found wherever pus is present – in surface wounds, eczema sores, for instance. The veterinary profession have themselves rightly pointed out that beta haemolytic streptococcus bacteria are themselves incapable of producing an acute condition in the body without the interference of other more toxic bacteria; therefore, as yet, we have no evidence to prove that the b.h.s. bacteria solely are responsible for sterility, abortion, fading of new-born puppies, death of weaned puppies, skin ailments, all of which are attributed to b.h.s. merely on the unsubstantial evidence that these bacteria have been taken in swabs from all such infected organs, bodies, or areas. The majority of the above symptoms can more generally be attributed to a general toxic condition of the animal body caused by long-term health degeneration of ancestors – and in the case of young puppy losses, of parent stock, the only remedy for which is, as in the case of the agricultural testament from which I have just quoted, not suppression of the symptoms by use of the highly dangerous sulphonamide drugs, but getting down to root causes, about which there is no call to repeat myself – sufficient to state merely the two words, *bad rearing*.

There can be no denying, however, that there are, in dogs, diseases of the reproductive organs very similar to the venereal diseases of the human body. Now many eminent doctors hold the rightful theory that such disease is mostly of a mucous or catarrhal nature, and is in part a self-cleansing attempt of the body. It must be agreed, however, that there is some degree of contagion, the disease being passed from stud dog to bitch during mating. But consider the large number of bitches which do have venereal infection – metritis is such an infection – entirely independent of any sexual intercourse whatsoever; maiden bitches quite commonly develop this disease. Though, even in contact with active disease, good health is an absolute safeguard, no stud dog could infect a really healthy bitch, and vice versa, for the bacteria must find unhealthy tissues on which to feed and multiply, and would very soon perish in the healthy alkaline tissues of the reproductive organs of a well-reared dog or bitch. Breeders, therefore, should not be too ready to blame infection on other people's stud dogs or bitches: let them look to the health of their own stock first, and remember that true health provides immunity to all disease, including worm infestation.

Professor A. Ehret, brilliant German professor of human medicine, son of a veterinary surgeon, author of many far-seeing English-written books on dietetics (on which he was an acknowledged great authority), has written words of much wisdom concerning venereal disease, which writings are completely in agreement with my own theories concerning such disease in human and veterinary medicine.

To quote from his writings:

There is no principal difference between any one kind of disease or another. In the case of venereal disease there is an exception, but only so far as symptoms of syphilis are concerned. Venereal disease can be healed by diet and fasting easily, for the simple reason that the patient is generally young in years. The cure becomes more difficult if drugs have been used. This unfortunately has happened in almost every case. The so-called characteristic symptoms of any kind of syphilitic disease are due to drugs of one or several kinds . . . Gonorrhoea. Nothing is easier to heal than this 'cold' or 'catarrh' of the sex organs, if untouched by drugs. Doctors must admit that the condition may exist without actual sexual intercourse, and therefore the germ can hardly be blamed. Gonorrhoea is simply an elimination through the natural elimination organ. If drug injections are used for any continual length of time, the mucus and pus are thrown back into the prostatic gland, bladder, etc. In the case of the female the entire womb, uterus, becomes inflamed, producing all kinds of typical women's diseases . . . Roseola or rose rash. A syphilitical eczema is due to the saltpetre-acid, silver-oxide injections. This is also the cause if gonorrhoea enters the bone. All are called syphilitic symptoms. Mercury is to blame for the hard chancre, secondary and tertiary syphilis.

The foregoing is of interest because it does well illustrate the harm done by the suppression of symptoms with chemicals. At present, the veterinary profession are mostly treating b.h.s. in dogs with either sulphonamide drugs or vaccines. If anything, the latter are less harmful than the former, for the damage done to various organs of the body by sulphonamides – especially to the kidneys and to the nervous system – is so difficult to remedy. Even supposedly 'simple' chemical tonic powers, in such wide use among pet dogs, may have a drug-accumulative effect in the canine body which is the cause of early senility, rheumatism, *eye ailments*, and many other abnormal body developments. The one and only cure for b.h.s. is a thorough internal cleansing of the body through fasting, use of harmless herbal medicines, and a corrective raw foods diet, all of which will remove the basic causes of the state of disease; cure usually takes from two to three months. But stock must not be bred from until six months following the satisfactory termination of the internal cleansing treatment. I have not yet heard of a single instance where cleansed stock have failed to breed normally.

A case of interest for streptococcal research work was an Alsatian bitch owned by the Templefield Kennels of Mrs J. Parr, Buxton. A bitch which for several years had been carefully reared on Natural Rearing methods, by Mrs J. Ixer, had been kennelled with other so-called b.h.s. cases. The owner of the stud dog to which the bitch was to be sent asked that the bitch should be tested for b.h.s. She was tested and found to be 'positive'. The tests were submitted to 'expert specialist' advice, and treatment with a course of specially prepared vaccine was prescribed for the bitch, together with similar treatment for all animals with which the bitch had been in contact. Ignoring such advice, Mrs Parr wrote me and, with Mrs Ixer's consent, it was decided to make a 'test case' of this Alsatian bitch. She was therefore mated to Mrs Parr's own stud dog, and has since whelped a perfectly normal litter, all of which were weaned easily. The puppies proved to be very healthy and exceptionally forward (always the case when the bitch has been given strict prenatal care with regard to diet and exercise). There was no doubt at all that the litter would grow up into healthy adulthood in the same way as so many condemned litters from other b.h.s.-diagnosed stock. In fact, a bitch puppy from this litter was a First Prize winner at the great show of the Alsatian League. The stud dog was awarded Best Dog in Show. It must in fairness be stated that the veterinary profession has itself issued the statement in the *Veterinary Record* and quoted in *Our Dogs* that b.h.s. 'can be isolated from the vaginas of most healthy bitches, so that its presence in swabs taken does not necessarily signify that it was the cause of the trouble' (abortion, death of suckling puppies, and sterility in the bitch).

In an effective article in *Our Dogs*, entitled 'The Worm in the Apple – Infertility', Vivienne Ferguson writes:

In addition to the normal hazards of keeping pedigree livestock of all kinds, another problem is causing worry to breeders. I refer to the problem of Fertility and the early death or even still-birth of the progeny.

This is a problem which has always existed, but there seems little doubt that it is steadily increasing and may eventually threaten the actual existence of certain strains or even certain breeds of dogs, as has already happened in different fields of animal husbandry . . .

Not Always the Parents. To show that not all cases of high mortality are due to faulty stock, I will quote an instance with my own dogs which occurred about fourteen years ago, and which was doubtless due to bad management on my part.

My bitches seldom missed, but though the puppies were born alive, seldom more than one survived to the end of the week . . . Despite skilled veterinary attention, blood tests, swabs, injections of various kinds and everything from the sulphonamides to autogenous vaccines, the only benefit was to my veterinary surgeon's pocket.

In despair, after resting the buildings, and thoroughly disinfecting everything, I drastically fasted my rather battered dogs (using the herbal cleansing method of Juliette de Baïracli Levy) and switched completely to natural feeding and management. One year later, my dogs, looking the picture of health, were rearing every puppy and there has been no further trouble.

Treatment All b.h.s. conditions, as in the case of venereal diseases of the human body, are infections of the mucous membranes, and are therefore largely catarrhal. Internal cleansing, together with most strict supervision of kennelling conditions, is the proved cure. *The advice on distemper treatment, i.e. internal cleansing* (fasting) treatment, as given in this book, must be strictly followed. But whereas distemper treatment is usually of merely three weeks' duration, b.h.s. treatment requires as a rule three *months* following the short fast to get the reproductive system really cleansed and restored to normal health. Reproduction is the most strenuous function of the living body, and if the body is unhealthy or drug saturated, then all manner of abnormalities can be expected in either the parents or the offspring of unhealthy stock. How breeders can deliberately mate unhealthy stock just for the sake of getting puppies to sell I really cannot understand; the mean things that people will do for money gain is an astonishing factor in human nature. One day it will be appreciated that the only true wealth is good health of both body and mind: 8o per cent of present-day domestic animals are unhealthy. To sum up: internal treatment is purely cleansing, followed by body building on a healthful raw diet; also a six-months' period of rest from all reproduction activity for both stud dogs and bitches.

Raspberry leaf, on account of its tonic effect on the organs of reproduction, can be used with great advantage for both dogs and bitches. Make a standard brew, and give a dose of the brew morning and evening for approximately three to six weeks. Average dose is two tablespoons morning and evening, or give in tablet form. For external cleansing of the reproductive organs, any of the aromatic herbs made into an infusion by the standard method are helpful – sage, thyme, rosemary or blackberry leaf infusion as used so successfully in eczema treatment can be used. Herbal compound tablets are more effective than the garlic for the prolonged treatment which follows the ten to eighteen days of internal cleansing.

Dog owners need have no fear concerning streptococcal infection. It is a disease confined solely to unhealthy, ill-reared stock, and is a natural result of overcrowded conditions. No well-reared animals can be affected. Keep small numbers of dogs only; feed them on the highest quality raw foods, give them the abundant free running exercise which their nature craves, let them grow up from puppyhood on clean grassland, then b.h.s. and all the other feared modern canine ailments cannot occur. In years of Afghan hound puppy rearing I have never given disease a thought among my own dogs, and stock of my 'Turkuman' prefix has been among the most eagerly sought stock in England, and has been chosen as foundation stock by leading kennels in England and America; the extraordinary good health of my NR stock was one of their chief attractions to buyers. Other breeders, concentrating on the rearing of healthy stock, have had the same experience and have found the same great demand for their stock. Health must be valued as highly as any show points; it is of higher value, indeed indispensable to the happiness of the dog and its survival and to the peace of mind of the owner also.

STUTTGART DISEASE This is a contagious disease which takes a rapid course and, if not treated immediately, can prove fatal. Symptoms are incessant vomiting and great thirst; the tongue often turns black. There is dysentery, sometimes with bleeding.

Treatment Treat as for distemper (see Distemper). Give an extra-strong dose of herbal antiseptic tablets or infusion of antiseptic herbs, which must include garlic. Treat the vomiting with gentian (see Sickness).

TAIL INJURIES The tail, especially the tip, often gets injured. The big breeds such as Great Danes and Irish wolfhounds are most prone to tail injuries when confined in kennels. They rap tail ends on walls and against doors.

Treatment Make a pulp of ivy leaves and apply, binding into place with a cotton wrapping. In between treatments with ivy, apply a salve of St John's wort. This herb of St John, pounded into lanoline, would suffice as salve. Alternative treatment is to apply witch hazel lotion. Also if available use sphagnum moss. Soak the witch hazel into the moss and bind into place. It is difficult to bandage the tail as it narrows at the end. Adhesive tape may have to be used.

TEETH The teeth of a healthy dog are a good example of what healthy teeth should be, in their strength and gleaming whiteness. However, a cooked or canned foods diet results in discoloured teeth and caries. Also when teeth are no longer needed for tearing at raw flesh and chewing through hard bone, they frequently deteriorate to the extent that in the modern dog faulty dentition has become a serious problem and a shame upon the canine race. Sometimes the premolar teeth are missing; they do not appear in the jaw as Nature intended to give the dog a complete set of teeth needed for a natural canine diet. Many dogs of many breeds now have one or two premolar teeth missing, usually in the lower jaw: they never came up through the gums. The absent teeth leave a great gap between the canine teeth and the first molars. The correct number of premolars in the dog is three each side, upper jaw, and four each side, lower jaw. Judges now penalize this faulty dentition among show dogs. The trouble can be hereditary. To overcome it, care should be taken in selection of breeding stock. Then there should be a return to natural diet, so that the daily food fully exercises jaws and teeth.

Treatment In tooth decay, treat internally as well as externally. For internal health improvement give such minerals and rich foods as: dried fruits (figs, raisins, dates), seaweed, comfrey, corn and oats, and raw marrow bones. Bathe gums with a strong brew of sage and rosemary leaves. Oil of cloves dropped into tooth cavities is a temporary pain-queller. Stained teeth can be cleaned by rubbing with charcoal made by burning wholewheat bread to black and then powdering. Apply with a soft brush and cold water. Teeth can also be rubbed with sage leaves and lavender spikes and with slices of fresh lemon.

THINNESS (See treatments under Appetite and Nervousness) Observe the case carefully for worms; if detected, then treat. It should be pointed out that most people like the domestic dog over-fat. The dog in natural health is, like the wolf, a lean, swift animal.

Treatment Increase rations of whole-grain cereal foods, feed some slices of buttered wholewheat bread daily. Give minced celery mixed into the meat, especially the leaves. Fenugreek seed is a great fattener and has been used through the ages to fatten horses. Soak the seed for twenty-four hours, using warm water. When soft, crush well and mix with the usual cereal meal. Also raisins can be fed in the morning, like pills into the mouth. Several dessertspoons early morning.

THYROID This is a glandular ailment. Treat as for obesity (see Obesity). Give especially all the iodine-rich herbs and foods: seaweed, garlic, egg yolks, raw. When available, give the great reed, Arundo donax, raw and finely minced, two teaspoons twice daily.

TICK FEVER This is more prevalent in very hot climates. The dog develops a fever and loses weight with alarming speed. Death can result.

Treatment This has been very successful and my herbal

treatment with garlic is well known in South Africa. Treat on distemper lines (see Distemper) with fasting and saturating the bloodstream with garlic, eucalyptus (a brew of the leaves), and other antiseptic herbs. For external protection against ticks, dust the dog regularly with herbal insect-repellent powder. During the tick season give sea salt on the food and increase the daily ration of seaweed; give bitter herbs in tablet form.

TUMOURS   (See Breast Tumours)

URINE, BLOOD IN   Bloody urine is often caused by a discharging abscess on a kidney, in turn brought on by a blow across the back area (over-common in dogs).

Treatment   Give drinks of a strong brew of parsley, preferably German parsley of the long thick roots. Keep on a diet of barley milk for several days. To make this drink, make a strong potion of barley water and add a half cup of this, tepid heat, to every half cup of milk. Sweeten with honey. Follow on with a light diet, beginning with several days on flaked barley, honey and white cheese only. A syrup made with rose hips can also be given.

VETERANS   (See also Senility) This state of life is, of course, not an ailment, it is the natural state of the elderly dog. Sadly, compared with man's, the life span of the dog is cruelly short, so that even if our dogs live to be over twenty years old (which can be achieved when there is good basic health and a careful and understanding human master or mistress) we are likely to have to bury three dogs or more in our own human lifetime.

The word 'veteran' can be applied to dogs over ten, although I have known dogs over twenty with the energy of juniors. The only special care needed now is a lighter diet, smaller and more tender bones to chew (now that the old teeth and jaws have lost their former power) and shorter walks, for it is thoughtless to overtire the veterans when limbs become less supple in old age, but at the same time it is selfish to neglect the much-loved and always needed walk. The veterans should be given extra attention in kind words and the showing of our gratefulness that they have stayed with us so long.

When the very old dog becomes 'troublesome', so slow of movement that the dog gets under our feet or becomes unable to control urine during the night hours, it is often a common solution to have the very old ones put down. One should think very carefully before ending artificially the life of any very old animal, be it horse or dog: so much kinder to let the animal literally sleep away into its natural death time. I remember my father's horse, Madralli. He loved this horse so much that he brought him from Turkey when he came to settle in England. In very old age the horse grew blind. He was given his own place in our garden where, in due time, he literally folded up his limbs and lay down in a permanent sleep of death. The old horse was then given a carefully marked tombstone and grave.

I like those words in 'A Poem from Ancient Greece' saying not to mock the dog's grave, for it was dug by a master's own hands and heavily watered by the tears that he shed for his dead dog.

Some more of my favourite words, concerning the death of an old dog, were written to me by Alberico Boncompagni Ludovisi, Prince of Venosa, Rome, who is a longtime follower of NR for his pointers and dairy cattle:

I am indeed much moved at your paying attention to my feelings towards animals – it was not long ago that my

fifteen-year-old pointer bitch died while I was literally holding her in my arms (for I knew the end of her life was very
near) and I could see 'the light' fading from her eyes while
sadly looking at me in a heart-rending farewell.

The soul leaves the body and then lives on, of course, as
you rightly said in your book – it lives on in more than one
way – placing all creatures, not just man, at the centre of the
universe.

VOMITING   The carnivores are natural vomiters. Just as the
owl performs regular internal cleansing through expelling
pellets of hair, feathers, etc, through the beak, so does the dog
at frequent intervals bring on deliberate internal cleansing by
eating things which will induce vomiting. In the vomiting,
excess bile and mucus and other impurities are expelled.

The most common vomit inducer used by the dog and cat is
that common weed couch grass (dog grass, twitch, crab grass),
*but the dog in its natural cleverness as an instinctive self-healing
herbalist* has a whole range of other herbal things which it will
seek out and eat to cause vomiting. I have observed my
Afghan hounds use all the following plants and tree leaves in
place of couch grass: leaves and stems of wild oats, maize
(corn), borage, goosegrass (cleavers), fig leaves. Big pieces of
gristle and bone are also eaten to vomit up much bile. Owners
of other breeds have told me of many more herbal things used
by their dogs to provoke vomiting.

But there is also the vomiting of illness, not caused by the
eating of specific things, and there is vomiting from eating
poison, from worm infestation, from gastric disorders, and
now from parvovirus.

Treatment   Cease all food except a liquid diet of barley water
and honey. Give drinks of plain water too. If poison is sus-
pected, give castor oil and senna laxatives, also charcoal

tablets, two nightly being an average dose.

To soothe the vomiting make pills of finely grated gentian root – any species of gentian – coating the bitter herb with flour and honey, or give in a spoonful of milk sweetened with honey.

A teaspoon of peppermint herb, sprinkled with a little powdered cloves and ginger and brewed in a tea, is also helpful as a vomit remedy, given as several spoonfuls three times a day; add a sprig of southernwood, if available.

WARTS AND CORNS Warts are usually a sign of glandular derangement, although they can sometimes be Nature's action of isolating body toxins beneath the skin surface. Do not use surgery.

Treatment The best treatment is internal, through diet. Feed plenty of raw minced dandelion leaves; also crushed boiled broad beans, given with the meat feed, are helpful. The best medicine, apart from diet, is seaweed powder, because of its high natural iodine content. For external treatment, the gypsies place great faith in the juice from stems or roots of dandelion or greater celandine. Squeeze out the milky-looking juice, touch the warts with the juice and allow to dry on. Apply the juice three times daily. The stalks of unripe green figs yield an excellent milky caustic juice for applying to warts. Also the white milky juice yielded when the skin of unripe papaya fruit is punctured.

WORMS This is one of the most important subjects in this book because more puppies and adults are actually killed or made permanent invalids through the mischievous and very common practice of worming with strong and irritant chemical drugs and purges than would ever die from the presence of worms themselves, or from any of the other common ailments of puppyhood.

I must begin by saying that, in spite of the advance in science, the subject of helminthology continues to remain 'wrapt in mystery'; what a far greater service scientists would render, both to humanity and the animal races, if they would devote more time to the study of parasitical worms, instead of spending all of their time and energies on research connected with Pasteur's discredited germ theory – that is, discredited by most thinking people. At present we know little beyond the fact that there are two types of worm which infect dogs: round worms and tapeworms, both types of which are divided into several varieties. And, further, that the ova of the worms enter the dog through the mouth, doing so from many sources: from infected ground (worm ova can lie dormant for years in soil); from stagnant, or even running water, to which other dogs or sheep or vermin – such as rabbits or rats – have access; from the milk of an infected bitch – in the case of puppies; from fleas which are carriers of a species of tapeworm, *Dypylidum canicum*, at which dogs bite, maddened by the skin irritation their presence causes; from worm-infested intestines of rabbits, cattle, or poultry; or from the flesh of such animals where the worm is then present in an encysted state. Cats are also common carriers of tapeworm.

It should be appreciated from the above details that if such a minute creature as a flea can be a host for a tapeworm, the larvae of the blowfly and other meat- and carrion-eating flies may well be worm-carriers also, as may be the flies themselves. Wild birds are often infected with worms, and domestic poultry very commonly are. The droppings of birds very soon dry into a dust-like consistency and spread over grassland, thus forming a very likely source of worms in dogs and other livestock. All this merely proves that it is almost *impossible* to prevent a dog, especially a puppy, from absorbing worms into its system from one source or another during its lifetime. But what is possible is the prevention of the worm eggs from ever developing into the adult worm, or, having developed, from breeding to an extent which would bring about worm infestation. The presence of a few round worms in the adult dog or puppy is no cause for alarm; as I shall prove later in this section on worms, their presence might even do good. It is only infestation which is harmful, and the only and certain way to prevent that state being reached is to keep the entire internal system of the dog, including the bloodstream, in a clean, healthy condition by means of careful and correct rearing, which includes hygienic kennelling and regular fasting. The presence of tapeworm is more serious than round worm, owing to the fact that the head of the tapeworm is armed with many hooks which attach themselves to the mucous membranes in various parts of the body, and these hooks may exert a harmful tearing action; while, further, the tapeworm generally excretes as waste matter a fluid which is an irritant to the dog's system, especially to the nerves and brain. But unlike the round worms, a tapeworm can rarely establish itself in a clean digestive tract, for it relies upon mucus deposits beneath which to shelter itself: the very presence of a tapeworm denotes unclean internal conditions. Though I must add that although the presence of a tapeworm in the body is known to cause some harm, it may also, as in the case of the round worm – which I deal with later – do a certain amount of good by absorbing a quantity of the sour food deposits and other toxic accumulations found in an unhealthy digestive tract. Tapeworm can create a big problem by establishing itself in a fold of the intestinal tract where it cannot be reached by the normally effective worm-repellent remedies. In this case it must be treated by diet. Following a day and night of fasting, give small, round cakes made of the following fresh ingredients: rue, wormwood and cayenne pepper (the hottest variety). One part of the first two ingredients and two parts of the pepper. Pound into fine

273

powder, then bind together with thick honey and flour. Make a tablespoon quantity of this mixture, press into small round cakes and press down the throat. After a half hour give a strong dose of castor oil or Epsom salts. I have cured the impossible tapeworm this way. Cayenne pepper for tapeworm was my own idea, but again I found that others had thought of it before me! It is much used by the Yemenite peasants for this purpose. Tabasco sauce, made in the USA but which has worldwide distribution, is a safe and excellent concentration of cayenne and can be used as above, made into pills. Dose: fifteen to twenty drops well mixed into flour and honey (for Tabasco is very potent) for an average size dog (tapeworm treatment). Ordinary worm prevention: a course of merely a few drops added to food, twice daily. Powdered ginger can replace pepper, or both can be combined: either or both are very good.

I need to classify here more definitely the types of canine worm, although there is no space in this book for any detailed descriptions – for such, a veterinary medicine textbook should be referred to. I will deal first with round worms, of which there are two distinct classes, although this fact is seldom realized by dog breeders. The type most generally found is the *Ascarides lumbricoides*, which again can be sub-divided into several distinct species, but all of which usually inhabit the small intestine, although when a state of infestation is reached they may leave their usual habitat and crawl into the stomach, or enter the bile duct (causing jaundice), or even invade the lungs, the nostrils, or the eyes. The other type is the *Ascarides vermiculares*, which inhabits the rectum and large intestines, and, in bitches, may spread into the vagina. The tapeworm family are classified under the name of *Taenia*, of which there are many varieties, but which cannot be clearly divided into distinct classes as in the case of the round worms.

(1) Round worms: Ascarides lumbricoides The modern veterinary treatment of rapid blasting out of the worms, with no regard to the sensitive structure of the digestive system, is not only useless but extremely harmful. For the health of the entire body is greatly dependent upon a sound digestive tract, and once the health of that important part of the body is destroyed by irritant vermicides – nearly all drug vermicides depend upon irritant properties for the removal of the worms – not only does the entire health of the puppy, or adult, suffer, but the weakened intestines become very suitable breeding-grounds for any further worms which may invade the body, and which will certainly then reproduce themselves in yet greater numbers in the weakened intestines or stomach which can now offer little resistance to the invading parasite. If the second crop of worms is removed by the same method, which method may even be repeated a third time, the resultant state of the dog's health can well be imagined. It is at such times that a condition of worm infestation is subsequently established, followed in many cases by the painful death of the puppy or even of the adult. It is also under such conditions that the disease-resisting powers of the dog become so lowered that one of the infectious diseases, frequently distemper or streptococcal infection, or parvovirus develops, and when the dog is seriously worm-infested its chances of recovery are then very slight, for the internal healing powers natural to every living creature will in such circumstances be but very feeble indeed. It can therefore be appreciated that treatment with potent drug vermifuges is worse than useless – it is killing; and such treatments are today killing off hundreds of puppies or, if not killing, permanently destroying the sound health which is the true birthright of all living things. In dealing with all types of worms the best treatment is preventive. In the case of puppies, commence this treatment before birth by disinfecting

the bloodstream of the dam (in which the worm eggs travel), and later the milk flow by the use of garlic. Then the correct rearing of the puppies on Natural Rearing methods, in order to ensure a strong, vigorous stomach and intestines, and healthy, pure bloodstream, the possession of which would never permit a state of worm infestation, but which would ensure the natural expulsion in the daily evacuation of faeces of any worms which have entered in egg form via the mouth and developed. But in the very usual case of a person purchasing worm-infested dogs, herbal treatment supplies safe and effective removal of the parasites.

Treatment, Worm Infestation Commence with a water-only fast of one day for a young puppy, two days for a puppy over six months or for an adult. Young puppies can have a little honey added, approximately one teaspoon per water dish, for an average size puppy. On the night of the fast give a strong dose of castor oil; one dessertspoon for an average size puppy under six months, less for a puppy under three months. A much increased dose for older dogs, i.e. one and a half tablespoons for an adult cocker-size dog, two tablespoons for an adult greyhound-type dog.

The following day, commence the treatment proper. A strong dose of herbal tablets, approximately six to eight, three-grain tablets, containing such herbs as garlic, rue, eucalyptus, etc, or other herbal worming tablets. Thirty minutes later give a further laxative dose of castor oil, the same quantities as above. Thirty minutes later give a warm, laxative feed of milk thickened with tree-barks' flour and honey, some flaked oats added. The meal should be semi-liquid. If the dog's stomach is very upset from prolonged worms, it may vomit this meal, which should then be newly prepared and given again after the lapse of thirty minutes. The tree-barks' flour acts as a soothing jelly which passes through the intestines, removing worms and their eggs.

Meals following wormings should be small, a cupful of liquid food for a six-month-old cocker, for example. Keep the dog on this fluid diet of three small meals of milk and honey, tree barks and cereal, for at least three days. A little whole-maize flour can be added, raw.

When the stomach and intestines are ulcerated from worm infestation, it is essential to rest them for a short period on a light diet of semi-fluid foods. Throughout the fluid diet give the early-morning dose of herbal tablets, but cut the dose by half, i.e. if six tablets were given for the worming, then reduce to three tablets for the morning continuation dose. Also, each night it is advisable to give a laxative of a mild and cleansing kind, such as senna pods. An average puppy dose of one large pod soaked in one tablespoon of cold water, with a pinch of ground ginger added to prevent griping. Senna dose for an adult greyhound would be four large senna pods soaked in the same way, using two tablespoons of cold water, with ginger added.

Now return the case to a normal diet, slowly introducing the NR raw food diet meals (see diets for puppies and adults, Chapter 1). Once solid foods have been restored to the diet, cease the night-time laxative. But add to the daily diet for some time worm-removing aids, such as grated raw coconut, grated raw carrot, ground pumpkin seeds (raw), cut seeds (raw) of nasturtium and of papaya, whole grape seeds, whole melon pips, finely chopped raw garlic. Do not aim to add all of these; one or two of these items would be beneficial. An average amount for a puppy of average breed would be one teaspoon of any one of them, or one dessertspoon for a cocker-size adult, given twice daily.

Also give two or three herbal tablets daily, average size dog, for approximately eighteen days.

In the case of puppies reinfecting themselves from sour

ground or ova-impregnated kennel floors or dirty yards, the worm treatment should be repeated for several days each month. Treatment is entirely harmless and is indeed internally tonic and cleansing, leaving the dog in better health than before treatment.

In all worm treatments it is a good thing to prepare the dog by starving the worm for several days before actual treatment is given. That is, do not feed foods known to be preferred by worms: fats, sugars, milk. Feed mainly flaked oats, skimmed and watered milk to soften the oats, and lightly boiled fish in place of raw or cooked meat.

Timing of Worm Treatment　The ancient people always recognized the fact that worms are greatly influenced by the moon. Worms become more active and commence breeding when the moon is waxing; they are less buried then in the tissues of their prey, therefore that is the correct time to plan worm treatment, when the moon is waxing, and then carrying out the actual deep cleansing with castor oil and herbal tablets *just before* full moon. I have well proved this theory in the worming treatment of dogs, goats, cows, and horses; the ancient belief, typical of many ancient things in medicine, was founded on intelligent observation by primitive man, taught by his own experience instead of from medical textbooks.

Alternative Worm Treatments　When the usual worming herbs as already given are not available, others may be used. Mustard seed: the seed is ground into a fine powder and given as worm seed. Average dose is one dessertspoon given in two tablespoons warmed skimmed milk. Or a mustard-plant infusion can be made by the usual strong infusion, using both leaves and flowers of the wild mustard plant. Follow the mustard with castor oil and the usual worming treatment as described above. Or green walnut leaves: make a strong infusion, two tablespoons of the infusion being given during fasting, followed by castor oil, or boil them in milk. Or six crushed green nasturtium seeds (average dose).

(2) *Round worms: Ascarides vermiculares* Enema treatments are necessary in addition to the above internal treatment as for round worms. A tepid solution of tobacco infused by the standard method. Or two tablespoons of the finely shredded leaves of the same plant, same infusion. In this enema treatment at least a half pint of infusion, for an average size dog, should be injected into the anus. Then, after the enema has been expelled, the anus should be bathed with an infusion of lavender or rosemary plant. As *Ascarides vermiculares* will also infect the vagina of female animals, vaginal treatments with rosemary or lavender infusion should be used.

(3) *Hook worms: Ancyclostoma caninum* When present to the extent of infestation, these cause a disease known as ancyclostomiasis, a form of severe anaemia due to the blood-sucking action peculiar to hook worms, which can even attack the muscles.

Treatment Same as for round worms. Treat also for Anaemia.

(4) *Heart worms* This worm finds its way to the heart, where it causes heart pains and anaemia. It is difficult to remove and often proves fatal; it is entirely mosquito-borne and therefore unlikely to be met in areas not troubled by mosquitoes. The life-cycle of the heart worm is complicated and very difficult to control once the development cycle has started. Therefore, the aim should be to *prevent* the first stage, which is the bite from the mosquito, by use of worm-deterrent herbs and by taking precautions against letting dogs have access to dirty

areas, such as public parks, or to boarding kennels where no good exercising facilities are available.

Another precaution is to bring dogs inside the house (or their kennels) at dusk, which is the time when mosquitoes are active. Bitter herbs in powder form can also be sprinkled on to the hair. And inside the legs powder with strongly perfumed talcum powder. (Talcum powder is suspect as cancer-causing. Ridiculous!)

When mosquitoes attack dogs and other animals, the bitten dog can take in the microfilaria which the mosquito is carrying in its sting apparatus. These microfilaria then undergo further stages of development while beneath the skin of the bitten dog, where they stay until they are strong enough to enter the veins in the skin. From there they travel onward until they reach the heart (which gives them their evil name, heart worms). Now they develop fast and can grow almost as long as two human fingers joined. Once mature, they breed and their offspring, the microfilaria, enter the bloodstream of the host animal, in which stage they await the bite of a mosquito to indraw them and carry them to new victims.

Symptoms A painful cough, distressed breathing, sometimes attacks of gasping, staggering gait, general anaemia. The orthodox veterinary treatment for heart worms differs, but almost all of it is poisonous and side effects are not known. My opinion is that these treatments, instead of killing the parasitical microfilaria or the adult worms in the heart, weaken the dog itself and so defeat their purpose. Indeed, the orthodox remedies advised are often worse than the worms for which they are being used, some of them containing such active and lethal poisons as arsenic or cyanide. Nervous disorders, permanent sterility, death from anaemia, are some results of common chemical heart worm treatments.

Treatment The aim is to maintain a healthy dog. It is well known that all animals have within them intricate and wonderful protective forces which control internal parasites, keeping them down to numbers which could never be classed as infestation and which can never actually kill the host animal.

Give salt and seaweed in the diet and dose with Herbal Compound tablets or pills containing minced rosemary, eucalyptus leaves and cayenne pepper or Tabasco sauce – average dose four tablets daily, mornings. (See also remedies under Anaemia and Heart.) Further advised herbal remedies are: thymol (extract of thyme herb), four to six drops for average size dog, given early morning in a spoonful of milk; and larrea (creosote bush extract) tablets, often known as chaparal, can be helpful. Chaparal is a strong herb so give two standard-size tablets four days a week, fasting, in the early morning, for one month. Then cease for two weeks, then use again, employing the same treatment for not longer than one month, every three months.

Whenever Herbal Compound tablets are not available, a rough copy can be made by mixing a teaspoon each of wormwood, sage, thyme and mint, all in dried, powdered form, and bound into pills with thick honey and flour. Pills should be approximately the size of an almond kernel. Three pills daily for an average size dog. Dried herbs are preferred because they are more concentrated, and thus more helpful in heart worms treatment. When wormwood is not available, its sister herb, the more common southernwood, can be used instead.

The American Indians intelligently practised mosquito control, through their bloodstream: *they made their blood unattractive to biting insects*. For example, during the mosquito seasons they would not eat sugary foods and they took into their diet bitter and pungent herbs such as celery seed, garlic, sage, coriander, southernwood, the strong-tasting berries, hot herbs such as cayenne, garlic, onion, ginger root. All these can be utilized for dogs.

(5) *Whip worms* Can penetrate deep into any areas of the body, including the lungs. Cause much irritation of the anus.

Treatment Same as for round worms. Give also anal washes using a bulb-type enema syringe. For the enema use any of the following: salty water, weak tobacco dust in solution (one dessertspoon to a pint of water) or a strong brew of cotton-lavender. If cotton-lavender is not available then common lavender, spica or vera can be used.

(6) *Tapeworm* This is a far more difficult parasite to expel than the round worm, for once it has established itself in the dog's body it is armed by Nature against attempts to dislodge it, the head of the tapeworm being provided with a sucker, and also a circle of hooks with which it digs itself into the mucous membrane, while it further protects itself by burying its body beneath mucus and other deposits which are invariably found in an unclean digestive tract. It is said in the East, by the Arabs, that only 'a foul body breeds loathsome worms', and it is further claimed that it is the partaking of cooked food – dead food – which causes worms. This opinion is, of course, contrary to the scientific fact that only by cooking flesh foods can the encysted forms of tape and other worms be destroyed. However, cooked food is 'dead' food, and means a general loss of health, and I myself have carefully proved that when cooked meat is regularly fed to dogs in place of the natural raw meat, worm trouble, especially tapeworm, is very frequent; no doubt this is due to the toxic accumulations from cooked foods which provide good breeding-grounds for worms, and thus encourage their presence. The harm that tapeworms cause in the body has been described earlier in this worm section.

Treatment   In tapeworm it is necessary to expel the head, for as long as the head remains the worm will continue to produce segments, each segment being itself a complete worm capable of developing into an independent worm. Treatment is primarily internal cleansing, and the complete treatment for round worm (*Ascarides lumbricoides*) should be followed. Garlic is a specific for tapeworm and has given excellent results, especially when combined with other antiseptic herbs. Dosage must be very strong, following the usual castor oil and fasting treatment (see Round worms). An average dose for the spaniel-size dog would be six three-grain tablets. Alternative herbal treatments are oil of male fern taken from the roots of the fern *Aspidium filix mas.*; this oil can be purchased from many chemists as it is still in use for human tapeworm treatment. Ask the pharmacist to prescribe dosage according to weight of dog; a common dose is half an ounce male fern oil mixed with half an ounce corn oil. One teaspoon of the mixture is then given after the usual twenty-four hours' fasting, with castor oil before and after. Also in use are areca and pomegranate. Areca nuts are from a species of palm tree and were once in very popular use. They are rather strong medicine for use on the modern dog with its weakened intestinal tracts resulting from unnatural rearing. But they are of service for the big breeds when herbal tablets are not obtainable. The nut contains an active ingredient, arecoline, which causes worms to loosen their grip on the tissue of their host. The nut should be freshly rubbed on a nutmeg grater for immediate use after the standard fasting castor-oil preparation, for the nut loses its value speedily after exposure to air. The required amount of powder is taken and mixed into a mass with thick honey and a little flour, using the tip of a dry knife.

Divide this bolus into several pills and press down the dog's throat. An average dose is a half teaspoon of the nut (before mixing) for fully matured puppies or adults of an average breed. Do not use areca for young puppies, in-whelp bitches, or toy breeds.

Pomegranate possesses an active worm-expellent ingredient, pelletierine, present in the rind of the fruit and more strongly in the bark of the root. The rind or bark, purchased from a herbalist, should be freshly powdered and prepared as described for male fern root, but no senna need be added. Pomegranate should also be used in conjunction with the fasting castor-oil treatment.

Charcoal, given in tablet form, is a useful addition to all worm treatments, when feeding is restored. Charcoal absorbs impurities from the internal organs, but it should not be used for longer than one month, with long intervals in between use, as it is apt to absorb too much from the body, including the good with the bad. The finely-sifted ash from wood-burning stoves and open fireplaces is a good worm deterrent and remedy. Put this out for dogs, in a basin, quite often.

WOUNDS (See Bleeding of Wounds) The advice given for bleeding of wounds should be followed; the dog or cat should be allowed to lick its wounds. When the wounds become infected, however, and also when there are many flies around (for many types of fly will lay eggs in wounds and they will develop into maggots, which can eat deeply into the body tissues) then use a different treatment which I have proved to be wonderfully effective. The treatment is equally good for human wounds and on two occasions I have cured gangrenous wounds by this Nature method.

I should like to say here that, if I have contributed anything truly useful to veterinary medicine, it is not only the use of fasting to cure sick animals, not the use of honey as a life saver, nor garlic and other herbs as supreme antiseptics, etc, but *this* treatment which I now give of the laying of fresh green leaves on to wounds, in place of the use of dressings and plasters.

Fresh green leaves, rinsed free of dust if necessary, are put directly on to the wounds and held in place with a cold-water dampened bandage. The preferred leaves are given in their order of usefulness: geranium (the common, smooth-leaved garden geranium is used, but remember that the wild plant, herb-Robert, in decoction, is esteemed one of the greatest of the wound herbs); nasturtium (big leaves), mallow, castor oil shrub (castor oil leaves are called *manus Christi*, supposed to resemble the hand of Christ, who used these leaves in his Natural Healing work), grape vine, hops. If none of these is available, the more common leaves of cabbage (inner), lettuce, or even dock may be used.

It will be found that the leaves peel off easily, causing no pain at all, and not tearing off scabs, etc, as in orthodox wound treatment, when ointments and plasters or bandages are applied directly on to wounds and the changing of surgical dressings becomes a most painful process and often damaging to the healing of the wounds.

Note: I had imagined that this use of fresh leaves was my own idea entirely, but later I was to learn otherwise. Some ten years after I had started to use the leaf method successfully for cure of wounds, a friend told me that the gypsies of Germany invariably wore a fresh cabbage leaf under a bandage on their wounds. Much later, on reading that lovely book, *Narka, The White Deer*, I found that when the white deer was seriously injured in a leg, the young Mexican boy who was with her took fresh leaves and bound them over the injury and continued the leaf treatment until healing was complete. Then again, much later and only recently in fact, I read in the book, *Green Mansions*, by W.H. Hudson (the story of primitive Venezuelan jungle life) of how, when a woman's leg was badly crushed, she was cured by the application of green leaves of a water plant. So I was myself only using and teaching something from my ancestral past.

Final Note: If your dog should become ill, and as a dog owner you have no experience of sickness, do send to a veterinary surgeon for his diagnosis, telling him firmly that you wish to treat the ailment with herbs. I am sure that he will prove to be both helpful and interested. Please do not write to me for personal advice. I have written my herbal book with its carefully-worked-out treatments for readers to carry out the treatments for themselves. I am away on my travels, and letters requesting veterinary help usually reach me months late, the dog probably having fully recovered by then; many do not reach me at all. I corresponded in former days when I was not travelling and could provide no detailed treatments in book form. Now I have this book which is fully able to answer all queries on treatments of most diseases in dogs.

PART THREE
General

8

The Failure of Disease Prevention through Vaccination and Hormones

Vaccination, although originated by the English country doctor, Edward Jenner, has been based largely on the germ theory of the French chemist, Louis Pasteur.

Pasteur was not able to keep his own body in good health and he suffered from paralysis of the mouth in his later years; he also lost, from disease, members of his own family. I have always believed in 'Healer, heal thyself first!' Then you have the authority to teach others how to heal themselves. If I had not been able to keep my own Afghan hounds, goats, hawks and horses in good health, I would never have possessed my absolute faith in herbal medicine and Nature Rearing, and would not have written my herbal books, or this present book, which brings right up to date my herbal work and gives over a hundred new and proven herbal treatments.

I have also watched my beliefs concerning the inability of vaccination to prevent canine disease come to be sadly, and overwhelmingly, proved correct. Disease rate among modern dogs has not been lowered by mass vaccination; it is greatly on the increase. Vaccination has produced numerous carriers of virulent diseases, or the treated dogs themselves, often given triple vaccinations nowadays, often develop all three of these very ailments – and die a speedy death.

The plague diseases of former days have not been controlled by vaccination; they owe their decline to those few benefits which man has derived from modern medicine, from improved sanitation and housing. Now vaccination is an exceedingly profitable business, both to the manufacturers of vaccines and to the distributors of these unnatural products: it will decline very slowly in popular esteem if it is ever allowed to die at all.

In an article entitled 'Statistical Studies of Distemper in Dogs', by Douglas S. Robson, PhD, there is mention of official study into vaccination failures and talk about necessary *annual* re-vaccination! Imagine that! The health hazards and the expense if large kennels accepted annual revaccination, all for a disease which is readily curable if it should develop!

That vaccination has an insidious effect on general canine health has been noted by observant dog breeders. It is one of the causes of chronic skin diseases, especially of the mange form. Also, greyhound owners have noted that vaccination has an adverse effect on the speed of their racing dogs. Mr James Baldwin, the well-known greyhound authority and breeder also of German shepherd dogs, wrote in *Dog World* concerning an anti-distemper-vaccination movement among Irish and English greyhound breeders, resulting from the adverse effects on the natural speed of their dogs, and in support of this he published a long statement from a greyhound man, whom he described as being 'one of England's most successful and experienced greyhound trainers that there has ever been' – giving his proof that vaccination made swift dogs slow.

In Switzerland and Austria many leading veterinary surgeons oppose distemper vaccination, declaring that it gives little protection and often undermines health; and in modern Israel there is very little canine distemper vaccine used, popular veterinary opinion being that it is useless and often gives the disease in a severe form to young stock who otherwise might never have the disease. I do not know of one dog in Tiberias, Israel (where I previously lived for many years), which has had canine distemper vaccination.

Personally I have no use for vaccinations whatsoever, and although during my travels my family and my dogs who accompany me are exposed to numerous new contagious ailments, the only protection which I desire for them is the all-round protection of good health resulting from careful daily diet of good, whole, natural foods, mostly eaten raw – as Nature intended for man and animals – also the use of disinfectant herbs.

In his writings, Dr Franz Hartmann, MD, a great theosophist, warns against vaccination. 'It would be interesting to find out how many chronic diseases and life-long evils are caused by vaccination.'

Dr Douglas Latto, MD, ChB, DRCOG, informs in his pamphlet, *The Fruits of Vivisection*: 'It is recognized that diphtheria immunization increases one's chances of getting infantile paralysis, and during an outbreak of infantile paralysis (*anterior poliomyelitis*) it is customary now to stop diphtheria immunization.'

The famed homeopathic doctor, Dorothy Shepherd, MD, condemning vaccination, has written: 'The more I follow up clinical histories, the more I am inclined to agree with opponents of vaccination, that vaccination instead of being a blessing has proved to be a wolf in sheep's clothing, and has produced more misery, more ill health, in its wake than almost any other method of treatment.'

There follow the opinions of two eminent doctors concerning distemper immunization; first, I quote Dr J.E.R. McDonagh, FRCS, the bacteriologist, in *The Nature of Disease*, Volume 1, pp. 75–6: 'Immunization with an attenuated virus cannot prevent distemper. The author has treated many dogs, which have developed distemper despite two or three injections of the preventative agent . . . He is of the opinion that fits, chorea, hysteria, etc, in dogs, have become more frequent since the use of Distemper Vaccine. Successful prevention will never be achieved by inoculation.'

And the other doctor, Dr W.J. Murphy – who 'before becoming a physician' was 'a graduated veterinarian' for fifteen years – expresses the opinion (which is absolutely my own opinion, and is now also the opinion of large numbers of dog breeders and owners): 'No serum nor virus for distemper is necessary nor can it accomplish any good for an ailment that has a natural tendency to get well of itself.'

Then famous people in the world of dogs have also given valuable and experienced opinion on this unnatural vaccination method of attempting to prevent diseases which come to domestic animals through man's unnatural rearing methods, which have shown no improvement or reform, but yearly increase in their unnaturalness.

Herewith I quote six opinons selected from the thirty which I published in the English first edition of my canine herbal book, which is still available in libraries.

1 LEO C. WILSON, journalist and international judge, writes in *Our Dogs*, England (1955).

People should not place too much faith in any form of inoculation against virus diseases since none yet discovered guarantees immunity. This is not to say that such inoculations are worthless but there is great danger that if people think that the inoculations do give positive immunity they are likely to take risks with their dogs which they would otherwise avoid and herein lies the pitfall.

2 CLIFFORD HUBBARD, international canine authority and author, contributor to *Our Dogs, Dog World, The Field*, etc. Author of *Dogs in Britain, The Observer Book of Dogs*, etc.

I have just read for the third time your book on *The Cure of*

Canine Distemper. I am completely in agreement with you on your views *against* the so-called immunization of dogs against distemper by the injection of various potent vaccines the exact micro-organism content of which must always remain unknown, and I admire your courage and sincerity of purpose in denouncing the orthodox treatment.

3 A.W. SALZMANN, chemist, Beudenfeldstrasse, 32, Bern, Switzerland.

Dr. Hermann Reitzer, of Vienna, has mentioned your veterinary book that distemper in dogs can be cured. Last year I lost three very wonderful Gordon Setters, and I do not need to tell you how eagerly I am looking forward to a cure. I am dealing already in serums, especially made to prevent distemper, but I am by now *convinced that no serum will help*. My dogs died of distemper in spite of vaccination.

4 M. MARCHANT, greyhound breeder, 142 Tickford Street, Newport Pagnell, Bucks.

I have great confidence in your distemper writings, especially as my mother who manages one of the Union Greyhound stud farms in South Africa, writes me that 50 valuable dogs were lost last year at their farm, all were inoculated. I cannot imagine why dog breeders should remain blind to the dangers of this orthodox treatment. I myself have had a favourite dog ruined by such treatment, and in a recent distemper epidemic two dogs survived out of 20.

5 G. MESSENGER, 10 Hunter's Road, Hockley, Birmingham.

I am in full agreement with all you state as to inoculation for distemper. The remedy is worse than the disease. You could not give me a dog if I knew it had been inoculated. The dog world owes you much for your exposure of this so-called cure; also for your real cure and remedies. I am no novice, having been breeding for 47 years, and exhibiting for 37 years.

6 GEORGE MUIR, P.O. Box 470, Place d'Armes, Montreal, Canada.

I have been very interested in your writings in *Our Dogs* on the subject of distemper inoculation and I have seen in the American *Dog World* that you have published a book on the distemper subject. Recently my interest in distemper has become very active, having just lost a very fine St Bernard female puppy two weeks after having the first of three inoculations under the — — method.

All those with whom I have since discussed the subject and who were in favour of inoculation, all maintained that the injections could not in any way affect the dog. Then they proceeded to contradict themselves by adding one or more of the following reservations: Don't inoculate during teething. Don't inoculate unless the dog is in perfect condition. Don't inoculate during Fall season (in Canada) as weather is so changeable. After inoculation, only exercise the dog but little for 7 days. After inoculation, don't allow contact with other dogs – 7 days. After inoculation, make sure that the dog is in no way subjected to draughts, etc.

Now why should all these reservations be made if the inoculation has no effect on the victim? The common-sense deduction to be made is in my opinion – inoculation reduces the natural disease resistance of a healthy animal – even although administered by experts; and who, in his own opinion at least, is not an expert?

I quote the following, without comment, from the American *Dog World*:

I had five German shepherd puppies inoculated against distemper. The veterinarian recommended and used the —— method. With each puppy we received an inoculation certificate. At a later date another kennel purchased these puppies along with an older male; the puppies were in good health. After they had had them for about one month, they sold three to individual buyers, and kept two of them and the older male for themselves. All of the six months puppies developed distemper and died, the ten months male, who was not inoculated and was kennelled in the same building, never acquired this disease. Are we in any way obligated to this kennel for the deaths of these puppies? . . . And *what is your opinion concerning the —— method*? (The italicizing of this last line is mine.)

And here is a further quote from a letter which reached me recently and was not meant to criticize vaccination; from Mrs A.M. Dryland, Bowenhurst, Church Crookham, Hants:

I have a Labrador bitch, and she was inoculated with —— against distemper and hard pad, as her breeder was very insistent on this. However, when we came here my bitch got distemper, and the *vet gave her an injection which he said would clear it up quickly and was the one used when a dog had been inoculated and had developed distemper*. (The italics are again mine.)

Here is George Hampden Edwards in *The Old English Sheepdog* quoting from my writings on canine distemper:

'For my part, using simple herbal treatment, including fasting, I have found distemper easy to treat, speedy to cure, and devoid of any after complications. Testimonials, world-wide, written in many languages, will uphold this statement.' But read the book for yourself. I am the more readily convinced that her approach to the care of animals, of the treatment of diseases, is the proper and best and most valid method, because I know it was successful in the past. Juliette has over the years collected the wisdom of the ages, before it slips away from us for ever. Over the years she has tested the value of the wisdom of old in the practical application of it to diseases. *And it is to her kinds of treatment that we must, in the end, return.* [My italics.]

Modern medical and veterinary science, however promising in some of its performances, is based on wrong premises.

INTENSIVE HERBAL IMMUNIZATION At such times as one finds that one's dogs have been in contact with other dogs suffering from any contagious disease, it is advisable to treat all immediately in the following way. Give them a one- or half-day fast, with a laxative that same night, and a dose of herbal antiseptic tablets last thing. Then daily give them Herbal Compound tablets every morning, or pills can be made from minced garlic, one drop of eucalyptus oil, wholewheat flour, and honey. Roll all the ingredients together and divide into pills – one drop of eucalyptus to every tablespoon of the mixture.

When known to have been in contact with cases of mange skin disease, bathe the dog immediately and rub into the body a lotion made of a standard infusion of rosemary or infusion of Herbal Protection powder, or rub down with a cloth sprinkled with oil of eucalyptus and spirit of camphor. Keep careful watch for three weeks for any sign of the disease and, if it should develop, treat as instructed for Mange.

When taking dogs to shows or public parks, give them a dose of protective herbs immediately before taking them there.

In Swaledale in the English Pennine mountains I had a memorable demonstration of the power of herbs to protect against contagious disease. There, in 1947, I saved around two thousand pedigree Swaledale sheep, condemned as incurable by orthodox medicine, as witnessed by many farmers. There was one field filled with seriously sick sheep suffering from a streptococcal infection, causing paralysis and blindness, and the adjoining field filled with well sheep, kept heavily dosed with herbs. Not one of the well sheep became infected from their sick neighbours.

In the late 1960s, Alberico Boncompagni Ludovisi, Prince of Venosa, Rome, Italy, treated foot-and-mouth disease with my herbal method. The cases treated recovered, and those immunized with herbal tablets (such as used against canine distemper, etc) did not take the disease.

TO NEUTRALIZE A VACCINATION SHOT Sometimes during travel when one comes to compulsory vaccination laws, one has to submit one's healthy dogs to the dangers and the uncleanliness of vaccination. When vaccination is to be given, take along a lemon cut into slices. Immediately the shot has been given take the dogs out of sight of the vaccinator and press outward around the place where the vaccine was injected. Then rub the area with the raw lemon juice which will help to kill the vaccine before it gets deep into the bloodstream. Semi-fast the dogs immediately, for at least one day, giving watered milk and honey only. Night of the semi-fast and the following night, give a strong laxative.

HORMONES These are a new and profitable development (for the manufacturers) in animal rearing. Each and every hormone treatment interferes with the delicate natural balance of the glandular system. I have witnessed so many health disasters and know of many deaths resulting from use of hormones, that I advise followers of Natural Rearing to avoid them absolutely, in any form.

Hormones are especially dangerous to in-whelp bitches. They are given for such ridiculous reasons as inducing a larger number of pups (breeders are pleased if they can thereby obtain fifteen pups in a litter, despite the fact that many of them will die). Often, freak puppies result, one or two pups of abnormal size, culminating in attempted Caesarian operation causing the death of the mother. Or hormones are given to check bitches from coming on heat, thereby causing them many health problems such as tumours in milk glands and uterus, loss of hair, often total baldness. I repeat, avoid modern hormone therapy totally.

9
Conclusion

I end my herbal book with the sincere hope that all readers putting into practice these herbal teachings will achieve for their dogs the same good health which has long been the possession of my own Turkuman Afghan hounds. Success in good health does not come overnight, it may take several generations to undo the bad health which man has been building up in his own life and the life of domestic animals during the past hundred years, when artificiality in medicine, diet, and agriculture began to predominate in the Western world. But success, in time, is sure, because Nature's own laws are unchanging, and Nature does not fail those who obey her simple laws.

As to the value of herbs – why should they possess the wonderful curative properties that I claim for them? The answer can be summed up in one sentence: they, the herbs, are manufactured by Nature, whereas drugs are manufactured by man (in the case of plant drugs, the normal properties of the plant are so destroyed in manufacture that there is usually little of Nature left in them). Now thinking people cannot deny that, try as he may, man cannot improve upon, or even hope ever to equal, the miraculous creations of Nature. Take but one example – the human eye: what an indescribably perfect thing it is, with its self-cleansing and healing mechanism, its remarkable powers of sight. Compare with the living eye the artificial glass eye that is manufactured by man. To that same extent there is in medicine the difference in values from all the products that are manufactured by Nature to those that are man made. The medicines in herbs are derived from the cosmic forces of sunlight, moonlight, and starlight; from rain and dew and the minerals of the earth's soil layers, as well as the hereditary properties. Any herb can have its medicinal properties analysed to a certain extent; only the cosmic and the hereditary cannot as yet be measured, which is unfortunate, for it is in this 'streaming spirit' of the herb that most of the healing powers are contained. Up to the present time little research has been carried out in connection with the cosmic forces contained in plants. Three men only have contributed useful knowledge on that subject: Dr Rudolf Steiner (the originator of biodynamic farming), Professor Edmond Szekely, and Dr Edward Bach and his famed Floral Remedies, remedies which treat the spirit as well as the body.

There has always been a great interest in herbs in America, and I feel that this is a result of the ancient Red Indian background. Also the Swiss are very herb-minded, and it is notable that my veterinary herbal books have gone into numerous editions in Switzerland.

One of my greatest inspirations in my herbal work has always been my detestation of vivisection. I am tired of the arguments in favour of this unnatural branch of unnatural chemical medicine, arguments sponsored by the vast sera manufacturing firms. The great and wise reformer of India, Ghandi, speaks clearly concerning this. 'Vivisection in my opinion is the blackest of all black crimes that man is at present committing against God and His fair creatures. We should be able to refuse to live if the price of living be the torture of sentient creatures.'

Mahatma Gandhi, in his deep wisdom, declared that the moral development of a nation can be judged by the way that they treat their animals. Believing this, one must therefore decide that the moral development of most of the so-called 'progressive' countries must be in great decline. I do not believe that any country in the world today has clean hands where their treatment of the animal population is concerned.

The very fact that humans will tolerate ruthless, modern factory farming systems, and buy the flesh or eggs from creatures so cruelly treated, is a wide black stain on all nations who permit and condone such immoral practices.

And yet more terrible is the condoning for profit of the exploitation of millions of animals of all kinds in medical laboratories and the manufacturing places of armaments and gases worldwide. Dogs, cats and monkeys are the particular victims because they react most nearly to humans to the experiments to which they are subjected. The beloved, sensitive, 'meek and mild' animals of the Bible – sheep – are now being used too.

I have never yet *seen* a laboratory dog or cat or other animal under stress in those places carefully barred to the public, carefully screened from layman eyes. If I were to see I should likely use violence to achieve their escape. But I *have seen* photographs smuggled out of such places, and I have noted the agony in the eyes of the victims. Although I have not seen the live laboratory animals in their prisons from which there is no return ticket (they are killed off when their usefulness has ended) I am tuned in to their wavelength and I do with every passing day feel and picture their pleading terror, their bewilderment, their anguish, and their waiting for the hope of escape. I am aware of their long pain: it has kept me at my work.

There was the need to prove conclusively that medicinal herbs are far superior in results to vaccines and chemo-therapy based on experiments on animals.

In recent years the interest in return to simple herbal

remedies has achieved a huge following. In 1982 the *Kennel Gazette*, the publication of England's ruling canine institution, the Kennel Club, printed an article written by me on Natural Rearing and herbal treatments for dogs, which they had asked me to write. The recognition had come eventually after nearly fifty years' work. One of the earliest followers of my work, and a trustee of the Kennel Club, was Viscount Chelmsford. He and his wife, Gillian, used Natural Rearing for their beagles, chows and dairy herd, with great success. Both were true animal lovers, and it was a pleasure to know them.

Modern man is astonishingly selfish towards almost all the animals he has domesticated. (The love and tenderness and care that the animals showed to the infant Jesus in the manger is all forgotten.) Modern man arranged that his factory farm slave animals live in soul-destroying boredom and hopelessness; many of them live out their shortened lives in small concrete stalls. They are refused the pleasure of parenthood (which God commanded Noah to arrange for all the animals of the Ark, 'two by two so that they should multiply') and deprived of this they are unable after death to survive on earth in the normal way through their natural offspring. Farm animals are now generally neutered for easier handling and for making more profit from the flesh of the overweight creatures which result from castration.

In the case of dog and cat, there is now a widespread practice, arranged for human ownership convenience, that is castrating of males and spaying of females. Such operations cause less household 'disturbance' at what would have been breeding times, less trouble from the dog going away from home in search of bitches, less 'mess' from the bitch when deprived by surgery of her twice-yearly menstruation cycle. I have written a booklet – *Against the Castrating and Spaying of Dogs and Cats* – in which I explain an alternative method of preventing unwanted matings, using a simple and totally harmless disguise-of-scent method.

The modern dog and cat often suffer deeply from daily boredom. Such boredom, because it is soul-destroying, can make normally kindly animals snappy and mean. Pets are left shut away in apartments for endless hours while their owners are at work, and the owner has little time on return home to give the sad pet the amount of exercise necessary to ensure both mental and bodily health.

George Hampden Edwards, FZS, in *Old English Sheepdogs* (Wentworth Books, Australia), writes about the cruelty of keeping adventurous-natured dogs on a short chain or in a confined space, and about modern boredom inflicted on a dog (linked to its need for sufficient exercise).

Altogether, the walking and racing about that dogs do is considerable (if unconfined) . . . I am quite sure that dogs need a great deal of hard exercise always. This is not only necessary for the body; it also dispels *boredom* which is an affliction we bestow upon all animals in greater measure nowadays than was ever the case in all history. This is the cause of much illness and disease, and it is particularly a part of modern factory farming.

I give now a quotation from a letter (also from Australia, where NR has a very wide following) which tells of happy dogs, and they are the breed I love, for their wild natures above all – the Afghan hound.

I used to be a vet nurse, for ever arguing over the advantages of NR versus chemical drugs, penicillin derivatives, etc. I have my own Afghans, and they run riot on my property. I have never before been a friend to such a wonderful dog as these Affies and I've never known such wild, lovable, primitive dogs as these.

When we lived in the Snowy Mountains – completely covered in snow in winter and a truly primitive area – our Afghans used to form a hunting pack and disappear over the horizon, swimming across the Snowy River, returning at dusk as the mists rolled: such a beautiful sight; and in winter their long coats would wrap round them like 'swank kinds' in fur coats!

– Deborah Fogarty, Tasmania

There remains in every human soul the love of the wild and the wilderness, and this feeling is yet stronger in animals.

Recently a book has been published entitled *The Wild Life of the Domestic Cat*. It is by Roger Tabor (Arrow Books, UK) and it tells in a convincing way how the domestic cat has retained most of its former wild-life traits and really continues to live 'wild' although sharing a conventional home with a human owner.

And what of the dog? Ah! the dog, who left the wilderness to companion man. I can write this for the dog:

I pray you who own me, let me continue to live close to Nature. Know that: I love to run beneath the sun, the moon and the stars; I need to feel the storm winds around me, and the touch of rain, hail, sleet and snow; I need to splash in streams and brooks, and to swim in ponds, lakes, rivers and seas; I need to be allowed to retain my kinship with Nature.

Dog owners, please remember these canine needs: they are for health as well as for happiness.

Humans should also try and retain that all-important kinship with Nature, such as the dog and cat still keep in their hearts.

I want this canine herbal book to encourage readers to collect their own herbal products fresh from the fields and woods, from the streamsides, the marshes and the sea-shores. Only do remember that since the first edition of this herbal book appeared many years ago the environment has undergone changes and we now live in a commercially poisoned world. So when we gather wild herbs we must be alert all the time to the dangers of possible weed sprays and drift from helicopters spraying insecticides which, unseen, can have made dangerous hitherto safe and beneficial plants: so gather carefully.

I shall always, despite modern hazards, continue to collect wild medicinal and salad plants for my own family and my animals: that is the least expensive way.

As for experiments in animal nutrition, I have been informed on several occasions that I must have carried out experiments in order to work out and prove my Natural Rearing diet method. No! Such testing was never required. Through mere common sense I knew that natural foods, medicines, and hygienic rearing *must* be best. I could never bring myself to divide a litter of puppies and rear one-half on healthy natural foods and watch the others decline on ortho-dox processed and cooked foods. I therefore reared all pup-pies by the same natural and healthy method – and as things happened it was other breeders who supplied 'controls' through their own orthodox methods of dog rearing. For instance, I have many times purchased, or had in place of stud fee, a young Afghan puppy from another breeder's orthodox-reared litter; that puppy, when internally cleansed and then put on to Natural Rearing, has developed into a strong, great-boned, heavily-coated adult, and has kept disease free; whereas other puppies from the same litter, kept by their owners to adult age on the orthodox methods, have developed into weak-boned, poor-coated specimens, and have fallen victims to the common canine ailments, especially worm infestation and the epidemic diseases. Well-known kennels throughout England, throughout the world, indeed, give testimony as to the superior health that Natural Rearing methods give in comparison to the orthodox, and unnatural, methods.

When I wrote my first article in the journal, *Our Dogs*, some fifty years ago, I warned against the health degeneration which would result if dog breeders persisted in the unnatural. Today we are seeing some of the tragic results of unnatural rearing. Because a cooked and canned food diet dispenses with the need for tearing and chewing, we find whole litters of dogs being born with the normal quota of teeth missing. The premolar teeth are not appearing in the jaw. Then, also through lack of Nature diet and sufficient exercise, there is the terrible affliction of hip dysplasia. This means ultimate lameness. None of these abnormalities is found in the wild carnivores, relatives of the dog such as wolf and jackal. Man's rearing has afflicted such upon the dog, and worse will follow unless immediate reforms are carried out.

The best preventive medicine remains true to the teachings of the ancient Greek doctor Hippocrates, who is considered to this day 'the father of all medicine'. One of Hippocrates' most famous rulings is: 'Let food be your medicine, and let medicine be your food.' And it is said of Hippocrates that he believed so greatly in the medicinal and food values of pure honey that one of the two basic remedies which he used for treatment of nearly all ailments was pure honey: 'hydromel', he called it, mixed with water, his second basic remedy was oxymel, honey and vinegar. Legend says that after his death at a great age, wild bees swarmed on his tomb and established their home there, and the honey taken therefrom possessed marvellous healing properties. As readers know, I have advised the use of honey as medicine and food throughout this herbal book.

The Greeks, and many peoples since, including the early American settlers, used to plant herbal gardens for use of their families and animals. Mr J.E. O'Donovan, of Eire, the greyhound expert and journalist, informed me, in one of his letters to me, that the old-fashioned Irish greyhound breeders very often grew garlic and other herbs for the use of their dogs. I know of several breeders in England, France, and Switzerland, who have already planted former kennel runs with those herbs which they have learned first from my books, and then second proved with their own dogs, to be of special value in canine diet and medicine.

Homeopathic treatments are presently popular as an alternative to chemical drugs. There are several books published in England and America on homeopathic treatments for dogs and cats. I, being purely a herbalist, have not used homeopathy, but I have heard of good results from this method and its remedies, and unlike chemo-therapy it is at least harmless and could do good. Numbers of qualified vets in the UK and USA are now using homeopathy.

There are also the teachings of Dr Edward Bach. Dr Bach invented Floral Remedies, which treat the spirit more than the actual body. I knew these remedies a near half century ago when they were yet rare, but nowadays they have had a long-deserved upsurge in popularity, especially in America. (Dr Pitcairn mentions them with approval in his veterinary book.) I have found them excellent for treatment of shock after an accident or following a difficult birthing or a bad fight among dogs. Again, these natural remedies are harmless and can give much benefit when used.

I am of the opinion that Pasteur-inspired vaccine therapy makes misleading promises. Promises are given that if vaccines are used against this and that disease there will be total immunity. The countless vaccine failures have proved that this is not a reliable contract. I do not want to make boastful claims for Natural Rearing and herbal medicine. There will be failures. The very nature of modern life invites a lower standard of health than prevailed in former times: polluted air and water, and the quality of the foods, be they flesh, cereal or vegetable, mostly declining in health values. Then this is the age of the machine, of the motor-car, and it is difficult to find safe places where dogs can run in freedom without risk of injury, and without exercise there can be no true health. *However*, when one chooses to be on the side of nature, one is on the winning side. Merely compare the health of the wild wolf and fox to that of the domestic dog, or the wild bee to that of the domestic varieties; there is the proof.

I now included a further paragraph from George Hampden Edwards' book about the English sheepdog:

> Let us not ruin breeds that have taken centuries in the making, either by following the geneticists' advices of short-cuts that promise quick improvements, or allowing our dogs to become guinea-pigs for chemical firms and drug manufacturers.
>
> [He then, kind to my work, continues]
>
> The best Vet you can possibly consult, and a Vet you can always have at hand, is the Baîracli book, *The Complete Herbal Book for the Dog*. That knowledgeable man of dogs, and particularly of gun-dogs, P.R. Moxon of the UK, has referred to this book as his 'canine bible', and I share his faith in the work of Juliette de Baîracli Levy. Her work for animals has been truly monumental.

I hope I can continue to merit this estimation! At least this latest, sixth, edition is a more complete book than the fourth edition to which Mr Edwards refers.

I would conclude with the quoting of some lines written by my friend, Mr L. Purcell Weaver, MA, concerning the naturalistic (cosmotherapy) medicine of Professor Edmond Szekely, whose books he translated from the French. For these lines are not inappropriate to describe the naturalistic veterinary medicine detailed in this book, which so many dog breeders are now resolutely following, and which kind of veterinary medicine is closely linked with the natural and true form of human medicine; and which, furthermore, has certainly met with much hostility and opposition. To quote: 'Its revolutionary teachings will be bitterly opposed in high places. It will triumph in the measure that it is true. And it is true in the measure that it heals. This can only be tested by each one giving the system a fair trial for himself and seeing the result. *Qui vivra verra.*'

I have always been a citer of quotations in my books because the cleverness of other writers gives support and help to the spirit which lives in every book. I have, therefore, chosen very carefully these two final passages to add to this new edition of my canine herbal.

The first extract is from that classic book, *Green Mansions*, by W.H. Hudson (Alfred A. Knopf and Bantam Books, USA):

O mystic bell-bird of the heavenly race of the swallow and dove, the quetzal and nightingale! When the brutish savage and the brutish white man that slay thee, one for food, the other for the benefit of Science, shall have passed away, live still, live to tell thy message to the blameless spiritualised race that shall come after us to possess the earth, not for a thousand years, but for ever.

The second extract is from *The Icelandic Saga* of Nial (AD970–1014). It tells of the Irish wolfhound:

I will give thee a dog which I got in Ireland. He is huge of limb, and for follower equal to an able man. Moreover he hath man's wit and will bark at thine enemies but never at thy friends. And he will see by each man's face whether he be ill or well disposed towards thee. And he will lay down his life for thee.

10

The Herbs in this Book

This appendix is for those who wish to gather their own herbs. Because most of the plants advised in the treatments are so common, no botanical descriptions are given, only the popular and botanical names, enabling readers to look them up in any book on wild flowers, where full descriptions will be given; botanical names are international and are the same in all countries and in all books of wild flowers, only popular names differ. As alternatives are given for many of the herbs in the treatments, those who cannot get one plant will usually be able to find another. A fuller account of these herbs and many others, and where they grow, and their medicinal properties is given in my *Complete Herbal Handbook for Farm and Stable* (Faber and Faber), in over a hundred pages of *materia medica* in that book, and herbal identification is provided in my book *The Illustrated Herbal Handbook* (Faber).

There are three lists: in the first are all common weeds, trees, or shrubs growing wild; the second consists of garden plants and herbs; and the third, a few herbs that must mostly be purchased from herbal shops. Nothing is said about the part to be used: that is given in the treatments, Chapter 7. Many health foods stores in England and the United States stock supplies of dried, plain herbs, suitable for canine use.

Once, when the first edition of this canine book appeared,

such shops were rare. Now one or more health stores can be found in almost every town in England and America certainly, and in many more towns worldwide.

I do not like authors of medicinal books to list their own products. Or I should write that I *did* not like it! But as the years have gone by I have learnt that this practice is often necessary, indeed is forced on one.

Take my own experience: I pioneered a short range of veterinary foods and herbal products which I evolved for use on my own animals and for my own veterinary work. I mentioned such formulae in my books because I needed them for my animals. Readers wrote and asked me to supply them. I did so and, without exception, users were very satisfied with the results. I did not want such commercial work: it kept me indoors, and I am wholeheartedly an outdoor person. But I could not reserve such formulae for the use of my own dogs and deprive others, so the herbal-formulae-by-post work continued.

Then, after some ten years, came a new development and a real challenge. Other people began to supply my exact range of products, one by one the very same! How could I know if such imitators were true herbalists and not just putting trash into *their* products (which can easily be done if one cares more for money profit than for the good of the animals using the products). Therefore, more than ever, I *had* to continue.

That is why my own herbal formulae are listed in this book and in my other veterinary books. It also gives me an opportunity to make known to new readers the other books which I have written for the welfare of animals of all kinds.

A director of a well-known herbal supplier in Canada, Joyce Rediker, Wide World of Herbs, Montreal, wrote to me quite recently that a person there was trying to copy my herbal products range (yet another of them!) and she sums up the true facts of this situation: 'I don't think you need worrry about it, since this person is interested in easy money with somebody else's effort; he is not likely to meet success.'

Wide World of Herbs can be recommended for sources of good herbs for Canadian readers of this book. They have not my own formulae available yet, but I hope to arrange this in the near future.

The more veterinary herbal products which become available, of course, and the more firms interested in developing this form of veterinary medicine, the better for the future of Alternative Medicine, as it is now called, but one would have more confidence in the firms who developed their own range of products rather than merely made a close copy based on someone else's efforts.

So-called Alternative Medicine now includes a range of medical treatments apart from the orthodox, including such fields as homeopathy (there is now a British Association of Homeopathic Veterinary Surgeons), acupuncture, etc. It is satisfying to know that the more that Alternative Medicine develops, the less amoral, cruel, vicious experiments on living animals will be used. As Alternative Medicine has clean roots, it does not work with dangerous substances which necessitate preliminary tests on animals in an attempt to prove their safety. The word *attempt* must be emphasized because we all know that many chemical medicines passed as safe have later been withdrawn by force on account of the harm they have done, sometimes provoking the death of their users.

COMMON WILD PLANTS

BILBERRY, WHORTLEBERRY (*Vaccinium myrtillus*. Vacciniaceae) Found on boggy heaths and on mountainsides. Its edible berries are well known.

BLACKBERRY, BRAMBLE (*Rubus fruticosus*. Rosaceae)   A common thorny hedgerow and wasteland herb, known for its juicy and edible fruits.

BORAGE (*Borago officinalis*. Boraginaceae)   Field and woodland, distinguished by its rough leaves and intensely blue flowers.

BROOM (*Cytisus scoparius*. Leguminosae)   Found on dry heaths and sandy soils. Possesses yellow, pea-form flowers.

CHAMOMILE (*Anthemis nobilis*. Compositae)   Waste places and damp places. Fragrant, small, daisy-like flowers; very scented, feathery leaves.

CHICKWEED (*Stellaria media*. Caryophyllaceae)   A tiny pasture herb with white, starry flowers.

CLOVER (RED) (*Trifolium pratense*. Leguminosae)   A common plant of pastures, with trefoil leaves and globes of red or pink flowers.

COMFREY (*Symphytum officinale*. Boraginaceae)   Inhabits ditch-sides, though will also grow in dry places. Now often cultivated as a fodder crop especially in Russia. Large, rough leaves; pinkish or creamy bell-like flowers.

COUCH GRASS, DOG GRASS, TWITCH, CRAB GRASS, etc (*Agropyrum repens*. Graminaceae)   A common grass of gardens and pastures. Has undergound, rather fleshy roots which are difficult to eradicate. Its leaves are long and very tough.

DANDELION (*Taraxacum officinale*. Compositae)   Common weed found on waste ground, on banks, and in gardens. Yellow flowers.

DOCK (*Rumex aquaticus*. Polygonaceae)   A common broad-leaf weed, with spikes of loose, rusty-coloured, reed-like flowers.

ELDER, ELDERBERRY (*Sambucus nigra*. Caprifoliaceae)   A small tree or shrub, with rich-scented, flat heads of creamy flowers, producing edible black berries.

ELDER, DWARF OR GROUND (*Sambucus ebulus*. Caprifoliaceae) Grows in waste places, is also a persistent garden weed. Resembles a small elder, but its leaves have a stronger odour and its flowers are scentless.

GOOSEGRASS, CLEAVERS (*Galium aparine*. Rubiaceae)   A trailing weed with round fruits and square stems, both of clinging nature.

HOLLY (*Ilex aquifolium*. Aquifoliaceae)   A well-known red-berried bush or tree with prickly leaves.

HOREHOUND (*Marrubium vulgare*. Labiatae)   Common in woodland and in hedgerows. Greyish, slightly woolly leaves, spikes of colourless flowers.

IVY (*Hedera helix*. Araliaceae)   A well-known evergreen climbing plant with colourless, sweet-scented blossoms. Found on trees, banks, old walls, etc.

MALE FERN (*Aspidium filix-mas*. Filices)   Likes woods and shady banks. Distinguished by its tall fern foliage which has numerous scales on the under surface of leaves, and brown spores.

MARSHMALLOW (*Althaea officinalis*. Malvaceae)   Of waysides, pink flowers, wheel-shaped, dark foliage.

MEADOWSWEET (*Filipendula ulmaria*. Rosaceae) Grows in wet meadows. Has rose-form leaves, plumes of creamy, sweet-scented flowers.

NETTLE, STINGING NETTLE (*Urtica dioica*. Urticaceae) A tall perennial, known by its leaves which sting sharply.

OAK (*Quercus robur*. Longaniaceae) A tree of woodlands. Has notable oval fruits in green cups, called acorns.

PLANTAIN (*Plantago major*. Plantaginaceae) Of pastureland and waste places. Distinguished by its flat-growing, oval-shaped and ribbed leaves, and unusual flowering spike, resembling a small bulrush, of greenish-brown hue.

RASPBERRY (*Rubus idaeus*. Rosaceae) A bramble-like woodland shrub, known for its juicy red berries.

THYME (*Thymus vulgaris*. Labiatae) Of moorland and sunny banks. Tiny leaves, the tufts of white-pink flowers of very sweet and aromatic scent.

TOAD-FLAX (*Linaria vulgaris*. Scrophulariaceae) Of pastures and waste places, distinguished by its yellow and cream 'snap-dragon' shaped flowers.

VIOLET (SWEET) (*Viola odorata*. Violaceae) Of shady banks and woodlands. Well known by its frail, fragrant, purple flowers. The garden species is also used.

WATERCRESS (*Nasturtium officinale*. Cruciferae) Well-known wild salad plant, growing in running streams, especially spring-water streams. If shop-bought, take care that it does not come from still, copper-sulphated water.

WILD ROSE, SWEET BRIAR (*Rosa* species. Rosaceae)   A well-known shrub of hedgerow and woodland. Distinguished by its sweet-scented pink flowers and hard, red, shiny, edible fruits – 'hips'.

WOOD-SAGE ((*Teucrium scorodonia*. Labiatae)   Of shady places and woodlands. Rough, dark leaves, spiky, greenish-yellow, hooded flowers.

YARROW (*Achillea millefolium*. Compositae)   A weed of lawns and pastures. Feathery leaves, flat heads of composite, tiny rose or cream-coloured flowers.

GARDEN PLANTS AND HERBS

ASPARAGUS (*Asparagus officinalis*. Lilaceae)   Known for its edible shoots. Also found wild.

BALM (*Melissa officinalis*. Labiatae)   Hairy leaves, whorls of creamy, hooded flowers; much sought by bees.

CRESS, GARDEN (*Lepidium sativum*. Cruciferae)   The common salad herb with 'hot' leaves.

GARLIC (*Allium sativum*. Liliaceae)   Early grown in gardens or bought from greengrocers. The wild variety grows in damp woodland and pastures.

HOLLYHOCK (*Althaea rosea*. Malvaceae)   Well known for its tallness and large flowers of various colours with squarish petals.

HYSSOP (*Hyssopus officinalis*. Labiatae)   An attractive, very aromatic border plant. Much celebrated in the Bible.

LAVENDER (*Lavandula vera*. Labiatae) Very fragrant when dry or fresh, has small greyish leaves and spikes of blue flowers.

LILY OF THE VALLEY (*Convallaria majalis*. Liliaceae) Well known for its sweet-scented, white bell flowers.

MARIGOLD (*Calendula officinalis*. Compositae) The well-known hardy annual of bright, orange-hued, daisy form or double daisy flowers.

MARJORAM (*Origanum vulgare* or *onites*. Labiatae) Very aromatic, of mountain origin, and resembles a tall wild thyme.

MINT (*Mentha viridis*. Labiatae) The common garden salad plant with mint scent.

MUSTARD (BLACK) (*Sinapis nigra*. Cruciferae) A common garden weed, with bright yellow flowers and strong-tasting cresslike leaves.

NASTURTIUM A semi-climber. Brilliant red, orange or yellow flowers with spur. Seeds in round clusters.

PARSLEY (*Petroselinum hortense*. Umbelliferae) Common garden herb, with flat or tightly curled leaves of intense green.

PEONY (*Paeonia officinalis*. Ranunculaceae) It has distinct solitary red or pink, large, many-petalled flowers, and large, fringed leaves.

POPPY (OPIUM) AND WILD, RED (*Papaver somniferum* and *Papaver rhoeas*. Papaveraceae) The former is a tall plant with grey-blue foliage and big, white-cream flowers; the latter, small, hairy stemmed with small, brilliant red flowers.

RASPBERRY (See Wild Herbs)

ROSEMARY (*Rosmarinus officinalis*. Labiatae) A very aromatic plant of grey-green foliage and small, light blue flowers.

RUE (*Ruta graveolens*. Rutaceae) Distinguished by its much-divided flat, greyish leaves, and small yellow flowers of bitter scent.

SAGE (*Salvia officinalis*. Labiatae) Popular garden culinary herb, also grows in abundance wild, on hills and plains. Grey, strongly scented foliage; spikes of blue flowers.

SOUTHERNWOOD (*Artemisia aboratum*. Compositae) Feathery, greyish leaves of intense bitterness. Flowers are small, yellow and flat discs.

WORMWOOD (*Artemisia absinthium*. Compositae) The same description as its sister herb southernwood, but foliage is coarser and of yet stronger bitterness.

HERBS TO BE PURCHASED FROM SELLERS

ELM (SLIPPERY), OR RED ELM (*Ulmus rubra*. Urticaceae) The pink-hued very aromatic bark is famous for its medicinal properties.

EUCALYPTUS (*Eucalyptus globulus*. Myrtaceae) This is a subtropical tree, distinguished by its tall, graceful form and willow-like foliage. The foliage can be collected in many parts of the Americas, but its extracted oil has to be purchased.

FENUGREEK (SEED) (*Trigonella foenum-graecum*. Leguminosae) Sold in some health foods stores.

LIQUORICE (*Glycyrrhiza glabra*. Leguminosae) The root can be bought from herbalists or the black solid juice (usually called Spanish liquorice) is sold in sticks.

SENNA (*Cassia acutifolia*. Leguminosae) Its foliage and flat seed-pods are sold by most herbalists and some chemists.

SKULLCAP (*Scutellaria lateriflora*. Labiatae) The dried herb is procurable from most herbalists.

WITCH HAZEL (*Hamamelis virginiana*. Hamamelidaceae) The bark is sold by herbalists, also its extract in alcohol. Most chemists sell the astringent extract.

PROPRIETARY HERBAL PRODUCTS

Natural Rearing products, compressed herbs in tablet form, especially 'Herbal Compound', garlic, rue, sage, wormwood, etc. Birthaid (raspberry, etc) tablets, comfrey tablets, seaweed with comfrey and cleavers, etc blend, and other blended powdered herbs and tree-barks' flour, also herbal insect-deterrent herbs, all made to my formulae, can be obtained from Larkhall Laboratories, Forest Road, Charlbury, Oxford, OX7 3HH, England (Director, Mr C. E. Woodward).
Floral Remedies from Edward Bach Centre, Mount Vernon, Sotwell, Wallingford, Oxon, England, or J. C. Nobrega, Av. Tomas L. de Victoria, VI Avda 141–1° Izda, E-43850 Cambrils-Bahta, Tarragona, Spain.

SOME HERB SUPPLIERS

Long established and with extensive supplies of herbs for mixing at home and on the farm.

ENGLAND Potters Herbal Supplies Ltd, Douglas Works, Leyland Mill Lane, Wigan, Lancashire, WN1 2SB; Fiddes Payne, The Spice Warehouse, Pepper Alley, Banbury, Oxfordshire

CANADA Wide World of Herbs Ltd, 11 St Catherine St East, Montreal, Quebec H2X 1K3

UNITED STATES OF AMERICA Indiana Botanic Gardens, P.O. Box 5, Hammond IN 46325; Nature's Herb Company, 281 Ellis Street, San Francisco, CA 94102; Penn Herb Company, 602 North Second Street, Philadelphia, PA 19123.

PREPARED HERBAL PRODUCTS

Prepared herbal products of good quality are becoming increasingly difficult to obtain. The problem is that destructive modernity has moved into herbs now that there is a worldwide demand for them, and it is likely to remain.

Formerly, herbal supplies were in the hands of true, caring herbalists, devoted gatherers who carefully air-dried the herbs in their own skilled way.

Presently, because herbs are now big-sellers, they are cultivated by the acre by quick-growing methods and are dried by electricity, instead of the former gentle way.

This quick drying by artificial heat turns the herbs an unnatural bright colour and renders them very brittle. The delicate essential oils, which are the main medicinal part of herbs, are damaged and often totally lost.

Note: To prevent evaporation loss, herbal pills need to be given a sugar coating to seal in their contents. (I am not an anti-sugar fanatic: a limited amount of sugar is harmless, and I prefer use of sugar to loss of essential oils of prepared herbs.)

Frequently I have purchased herbs by post and, on opening the packets, have thrown the herbs out into my garden because for medicinal purposes they were useless, without proper colour and scent. Among such throwouts was an expensive purchase of French lavender. France was once famed for its lavender: the growers will have to return to natural drying if they want to keep their good name.

Therefore, one must be very careful as to what quality of herbs are going into commercial products. This also concerns my own fomulae because in the past some former suppliers have broken faith and used substandard herbs and added chemicals to my recommended recipes.

When there is difficulty in obtaining high-grade herbal products by post, learn to make home remedies. One does not want one's animals to be deprived of important herbal help because some people are exploiting them for commercial gain. One gives time to preparing daily food for one's family, so some time can be given to preparing food for the animals. It does not take long to mix up some dried, powdered herbs and bind them into pills with flour and thick honey.

My basic advice for home-made remedies is not to use the very potent herbs, even though I recommend them in my books: they are for the experienced.

Substitute milder herbs instead.

Rue and wormwood are both very potent herbs – leave them out (though I love them both). Rue can be replaced by vervain or marjoram, and wormwood by the milder southernwood (of the same family). For *external* use, rue and wormwood are both appropriate, no precise prescribing being needed.

A home mixture for deterring skin pests can easily be made, in lotion or soaked in hot oil, to treat sores and wounds; any of the wounds and skin treatment herbs mentioned in this book, all in equal amounts. Such herbs would include southernwood or wormwood, sage, rosemary, vervain, marjoram, nasturtium (especially the seeds), all types of mint; if being used in dry powder form, for bulk add powdered barks of eucalyptus and any type of pine tree.

11

Recommended Reading

Dr Pitcairn's Complete Guide to Natural Health for Dogs and Cats, Richard H. Pitcairn, DVM, PhD, and Susan Hubble Pitcairn (Rodale Press, USA, 1982). The book praises the Baîracli herbal veterinary work. Homeopathy is also dealt with extensively.

The Mastiff and Bullmastiff Handbook, D.B. Oliff (Boydell & Brewer, UK; Howell Book House Inc., USA). A careful and detailed book on the mastiff. The author was one of the first canine breeders to adopt Natural Rearing.

The Afghan Hound: A Definitive Study, Margaret Niblock (K & R Books Ltd). The greatest of the Afghan books. Includes a chapter on Natural Rearing by J. de B.L. Now obtainable only from the author, price £25. Niblock, Barnard Gate Farm, Barnard Gate, Nr Witney, Oxon, England.

Old English Sheepdogs in Australia, George Hampden Edwards, FZS (Wentworth Books, Australia). Based on forty years' association with the breed in Australia and abroad. Successes with Natural Rearing and herbal veterinary treatment are given.

Talking to Animals, Barbara Woodhouse (Penguin). This deservedly famous book is not associated with Natural

Rearing, although the author did give natural care to her many animals. It is recommended because deep love for animals is found throughout and dogs and cats are, of course, included.

A NOTE FROM THE AUTHOR

I sincerely regret that it is no longer possible to answer readers' veterinary problems sent to me in the post. Because I travel so much, months often go by without mail reaching me and very many letters are lost as a result of my being out of reach of mail.

I have again, for this new edition of the *Complete Herbal Handbook for the Dog and Cat*, studied carefully all the treatments given to make sure that all can be followed with ease and without needing any help from myself.

Of course there will be many ailments not dealt with in this book, which gives only the more general ones. To include all known ailments would make my book such a lengthy one that it would no more be a useful handbook, but would become a heavy tome too highly priced for most smallholders and farmers to care to buy and use.

Furthermore, this book is in many foreign translations, in addition to the British and American editions, and if all those countless thousands who now have a copy of it were to write to me for personal advice, my every day and most of every night would be fully taken in writing letters. Impossible! Nor can I, in fairness, answer a few chosen persons and not answer all. Unjust. Again impossible!

I have had a deep love for animals from early childhood to my present age, which has now reached the official one of retirement from work. I know that I can best serve animals by practical study of their needs in the field, during my continuing travels, and not monotonously, and *unwillingly*, confined to a room with a typewriter. Therefore, please do not write to me. I thank you for reading this book, all the thousands of you – 40,000 in America, for happy example – and I know that it will help your animals, as it has helped mine.

Indexes

General Index

In all three indexes, where the first one or two numbers are out of ascending order these are the main reference

Index of Ailments

Materia Medica Botanica

341